CHANCE FOR CHANGE

*Implications of a Chronic
Disease Module Study*

CHANCE FOR CHANGE
Implications of a Chronic Disease Module Study

edited by　Joseph A. Papsidero
Sidney Katz
Sr. Mary Honora Kroger, R.S.M.
C. Amechi Akpom

Michigan State University Press, East Lansing, Michigan

Manufactured in the United States of America

DEDICATION

This book is dedicated to Margaret Blenkner D.S.W., brilliant, compassionate teacher, social worker, and research methodologist. Her techniques and experimental studies in social work and public health nursing services have had a wide impact on care of the aged and have received national and international recognition.

Dr. Blenkner, Project Director for the Chronic Disease Module Project from its inception in 1972 until her death in August 1973, brought to the project a unique depth of vision and grasp of research which she expertly applied in collaboration with the principal and co-principal investigators.

CONTENTS

PREFACE

During the present century, radical changes have taken place in the population age structures of developed countries. This has changed the nature of health problems that confront the health services systems of these countries. Leading causes of death and disability have shifted from acute infectious diseases, which affect the first part of the lifespan, to the chronic diseases, which increase steadily after early adulthood. Increasingly thrust upon our attention are the problems generated by chronic illnesses and disabilities. It is clear that at this time in our country, existing health services cope with such health problems in a discontinuous and fragmented way. For the disabled person at home, services tend to become even more remote and episodic. Although help is clearly needed, few of our communities are prepared to meet even simple needs of chronically ill persons who live at home.

At the same time as the needs of the chronically ill demand more attention, major social forces in the United States challenge us to meet these needs through services that are appropriately accessible, available, efficient, and effective. One result of these social forces has been a search for alternative approaches to the delivery of care. For the care of chronically ill and aging people, the alternative of home care has been "rediscovered." It is being redefined in emerging health policy and through programmatic changes in the financing, organization, and delivery of health services.

This book aims to contribute to the knowledge and experimental base required for rational policy and program decisions. It is based upon a five-year demonstration and evaluation program conducted between 1971 and 1976. The aim of the program was to evaluate the effects of an interdisciplinary team approach to home care, utilizing a new type of health assistant. The concept of care upon which this program was based was derived from research systematically conducted by Sidney Katz and his associates over the past fifteen years. In particular, the study described in this book is a logical extension of a controlled longitudinal study that was described in *Effects of Continued Care* authored by Sidney Katz and others.

The goals and objectives of our Chronic Disease Module study as reported here are, first, placed in a social perspective wherein current and emerging long-term care directions and policy are identified. After a literature review of relevant issues and problems, an overview of the major features of the study design and methods is presented. This is followed by a description of organizational, community, and population characteristics of each setting in the study. Described next are the functional and operational elements of the service that was delivered by home care teams, which we called "Chronic Disease Modules." The results of the study are then presented and the book concludes with a discussion of these results in terms of their implications for public policy.

Service program managers, planners, and policy-makers should find this book useful. It should also be useful to practitioners, providers, and students in the health professions.

ACKNOWLEDGMENTS

Grateful acknowledgment is made of all those who directly or indirectly participated in this study. Although it is not possible to list the names and contributions of the 874 participants; the eleven persons who served on the Executive Committee; the forty-five staff members; the fourteen resource persons; the thirty-eight members of the module staffs; the twenty-one members of the evaluation field unit staff; the twenty-five research and training consultants; the five participating community colleges; and the twenty-three participating host agencies and referral sources who made the Chronic Disease Module project possible, our appreciation and indebtedness are nevertheless expressed.

This book is based on work performed pursuant to research grant HS01059 from the National Center for Health Services Research, Department of Health, Education and Welfare.

Chapter 1

INTRODUCTION:
THE SOCIAL SCENE

Sidney Katz

The 20-year period that followed the Second World War witnessed the results of increasing social concern throughout the world. By 1964, more than 100 countries had social security programs, and 82 had sickness and/or maternity benefits (DHEW 1964). In the United States as well, people increasingly applied their economic and political strength to develop solutions for health and welfare problems. A subset of these problems is that of meeting the needs of the growing number of citizens disabled by age and illness. For these citizens, the passage of Medicare in the Social Security Amendments Act of 1965 was a particularly important event (U.S. Congress 1965) which translated social concern into social action. This action recognized that nonpublic approaches had not met the needs of our affected fellow citizens, and that the responsibility was a public obligation. Medicare thus served as an instrument that expressed health-related values as national policy. In a major and unpredictable manner, it influenced the subsequent development of our health and welfare system, our economic system, and even our processes of government. Medicare opened the door to expanded public financing of health services, to publicly directed changes in the organization and delivery of health services, and to public accountability for standards of services.

As evidence of the forces set in motion by Medicare, we need only examine the many national directions that have emerged. For long-term care of disabled people these directions are reflected in legislation such as the Social Security Amendments Act of 1972, the Health Maintenance Organization Act of 1973, the National Health Planning and Resources Development Act of 1974, and proposed national health insurance of 1975. In the Social Security Amendments Act of 1972, Congress provided for the establishment of the Professional Standards Review Organization Program (PSRO). Its purpose is to assess and improve the quality of health care for Federal beneficiaries through local organizations (U.S. Congress 1972). For large segments of our disabled population, the currently fragmented system of health services does not adequately meet multidisciplinary and continuous needs. Quality assurance for the disabled is thus a function of each separate individual or organization that provides services. Such quality assurance can only be fragmented and uncertain—both in concept and practice. As a unique social development, PSRO legislation represents the introduction of public accountability for standards of service and represents a stimulus to develop non-fragmented services for the disabled.

Current Health Maintenance Organization (HMO) legislation seeks to improve the continuity of care and emphasizes ambulatory and preventive care (U.S. Congress 1973). This legislation requires that long-term care be provided through a services package that includes services in intermediary and long-term facilities, physical medicine and rehabilitation services, and home health services. Responsibility is thus assumed for a broad spectrum of problems of the disabled and chronically ill. For these people, decreased socioeconomic productivity and worsening of the quality of life are often serious consequences of their decreased physical, psychological, and social functioning. The associated dependencies also become problems to the family and community. The preventive and comprehensive care orientation of HMO legislation requires that we address these problems, that we interrupt or slow down deteriorating function where we can, and that we minimize its negative effect on the quality of life. In response to legislation, we see the emergence of changes in the organization and delivery of long-term care, as well as new technologies and new information and evaluation systems.

As one important manifestation of the forces moving to change the organization and delivery of care, the National Health Planning and Resources Development Act of 1974 aims to integrate and improve our planning, regulatory, and resource distribution efforts (U.S. Congress 1974). Planning agencies under this act have functions designed to address issues of access, cost, and resource allocation. They also have clear roles in the regulatory decision-making process—as, for example, in certificate-of-need decisions. Through this planning legislation, we are required to deal with problems associated with the increasing cost of care and the major commitment of resources needed for long-term care. We are asked to direct our attention to approaches that integrate the basic living supports and multidisciplinary elements of service that make up long-term care. We are asked to emphasize the continuous and nonepisodic aspects of such care in a humane, effective, and socially responsible manner. Even as we stress continuity, we are asked to avoid inappropriate dependence on services and to provide for discontinuance of unnecessary services. This planning legislation represents a significant step toward public involvement in changing the organization and delivery of long-term care.

Not the least of the evidence of strong social forces in current national directions is the continuing development of legislation for national health insurance (DHEW 1975). The goal of this effect is to improve health care financing and to assure that every person has the opportunity to receive needed health care services. A comprehensive program of national health insurance would extend the opportunity for long-term services to disabled people. It would facilitate elimination of a multitiered system that discriminates especially against disabled, disadvantaged people. In view of the significant public and legislative constituency that supports it, national health insurance is needed to eliminate the fragmented nature of services for the disabled.

The foregoing legislation and related activities reflect emerging public policy and the instruments through which such policy is to be implemented. The social forces that call for implementation have pressed us to make decisions and to take action. Often, such effort has lacked the adequate information base that would make our planning, programs, and processes sufficiently rational. As a result, we have made, and continue to make, serious and costly mistakes that delay aid for those who suffer. Adequate information is not available, for example, about needs, outcomes that should and could be expected as a result of services, or the nature of the services themselves. From an organizational viewpoint, missing information about problems, processes, outcomes, and costs is a barrier to rational planning for the structure of service programs, as well as for their funding, administration, and monitoring. From a service viewpoint, we need such information to define the appropriate targets for service, as well as the type of service, and the necessary manpower. The rational evolution of policy also requires such information.

Although Medicare financed expanded opportunities for service, we were not prepared for the increased administrative burdens and costs. Costs also were higher as a result of greater service usage that initially increased hospital occupancy and decreased the amount of free care given (Feldstein 1968). Although the financial position of hospitals improved, we did not know whether the increased services and costs had improved care (Teeling-Smith 1973). We faced the fact that more money is not synonymous with better care and that all treatment is not necessarily beneficial; yet we lacked the information and ability to deal with such issues. We recognized the need to incorporate quality assurance systems, and we legislated through PSRO to implement assurance mechanisms. Thereupon, we found ourselves in the position of lacking significant information about the impact of services on disabilities and chronic illnesses that consume major amounts of resources. As a result, we concentrated our quality assurance efforts on the development of expensive organizations, information technologies, and process criteria without adequate attention to the assessment of patient outcomes. Our costly efforts were not, in fact, implementation activities. They were largely exploratory and developmental activities. Relatedly, we enacted laws to plan and organize for better health care systems—namely, the laws that established Regional Medical Programs and Comprehensive Health Planning. These efforts floundered since we were not as ready to implement better health care systems as many had assumed. We became increasingly aware of the inadequacy of available information for sound planning. Subsequently we reorganized our efforts through the National Health Planning and Resources Development Act, in which the mandate for the development and use of sound information was expressed clearly. With regard to the continuing development of legislation for national health insurance, we cannot adequately estimate such important dimensions as the demand for services that will emerge, the manpower requirements (i.e., supply), and the supply response. We thus again face the serious likelihood of costly errors in decisions.

The significance of the study reported in this book is related to its ability to contribute useful information to the policy-making and planning activities represented in the previously described national directions. The study concerns the acceptance and impact of care delivered to disabled people at home by a small team of providers, including supervised health assistants. In our earlier book, *The Effects of Continued Care* (Katz, et al. 1972) we reported the results of a study designed to find out whether the planned use of one available method of coordinating and continuing health services—namely, continuing home visits by a public health nurse, working with the patient's physician and with community resources —could improve or maintain the function of a group of disabled patients who were fifty years or older and who lived at home. In this earlier controlled study, two years of services were given to randomly selected, chronically ill patients who were discharged from a hospital for the chronically ill. Outcomes in the treated group were compared with outcomes in randomly selected patients who were not assigned to the service program. Observations of outcome were made by observers who were functionally and geographically separated from the people who provided services.

The earlier study showed that the less disabled, less severely ill patients who received the home service program tended to experience more physical and psychological benefits than comparable patients in the control group. Those who were younger benefited similarly, as did those who functioned adequately mentally and those who had uncomplicated musculoskeletal disease. Older patients who received the home service program used more community health services than comparable patients in the control group, without showing measurable functional benefits, as did those with central nervous system or cardiovascular disease. Quantitative estimates were made of the benefits, differences in social functioning, and use of services. As one example of such quantitative estimates, the study showed that approximately half the patients with arthritis who were assigned to the home service program maintained limb movement that they would have lost had they not received this care. Thus, the study contributed specific information about the outcomes of the home service program.

As a result of the earlier findings, we conducted the study reported here, in which we made available a less costly alternative—namely, a program of continuing home visits by health assistants. These health assistants were given responsibilities for the care of the chronically ill and worked as part of a small team directed by professionals. This service was made available to people who needed less than skilled professional care. In an experimental demonstration, we evaluated the acceptance, outcome, and costs of the new alternative in actual community settings. We were interested in the following questions: Would the findings of the earlier, rigorous experiment be supported? How useful would the service be as a product of three interwoven factors: acceptance, effectiveness, and cost? What new insights beyond the prior study would we gain into the nature of continuing community care? What implications would our findings have for long-term care policy development and implementation by legislators, planners, and regulators? What implications would the findings have for guidelines related to the management of service programs for aging and chronically ill people? In this book, we describe the study and its results in order to shed what light we can on these questions.

REFERENCES

Feldstein, P. and Waldman, S. 1968. Financial position of hospitals in early Medicare period. *Social Security Bulletin* 31:18–23.

Katz, S., Ford, A. B., Downs, T. D., Adams, M., and Rusby, D. I. 1972. *Effects of Continued Care: A Study of Chronic Illness in the Home.* DHEW Publication No. (HSM) 73–3010. U.S. Government Printing Office, Washington, D.C., pp. 76–82.

Teeling-Smith, G. 1973. More money into the medical sector: Is this the answer? *International Journal of Health Services* 3:493–500.

U.S. Congress. 1965. *Public Law 89–97, Medicare, Title 18 of the Social Security Amendments Act of 1965.* Washington, D.C.

U.S. Congress. 1972. *Public Law 92–603, Social Security Amendments Act of 1972.* Washington, D.C.

U.S. Congress. 1973. *Public Law 93–222, Health Maintenance Organization Act, Part 110.* Washington, D.C.

U.S. Congress. 1974. *Public Law 93–641, National Health Planning and Resources Development Act.* Washington, D.C.

U.S. Department of Health, Education, and Welfare. 1975. *Forward Plan for Health FY1977–81.* DHEW Publication No. (OS) 76–50024. U.S. Government Printing Office, Washington, D.C.

U.S. Department of Health, Education, and Welfare. Social Security Administration. Division of Research and Statistics. 1964. *Social Security Programs Throughout the World 1964.* U.S. Government Printing Office, Washington, D.C.

Chapter 2

RELEVANT ISSUES
AND DEVELOPMENTS

Sister Mary Honora Kroger
Joseph Papsidero

The health care needs of the chronically ill aged, programs to meet these needs, and the effectiveness and efficiency of such programs are socially important concerns. They have been topics of growing interest and concern to health care providers, social gerontologists, and public agencies in recent years. This chapter reviews the major issues related to these concerns which are addressed in our study. These issues will be discussed in four sections: problems of the chronically ill aged, home care programs for the chronically ill, new health care manpower, and interdisciplinary team care.

PROBLEMS OF THE CHRONICALLY ILL

With advancing years, the health of most people deteriorates. Chronic conditions such as heart disease and arthritis become far more prevalent. The three leading causes of death among the elderly—heart disease, cancer, and cerebrovascular disease—require large quantities of health care services. They may also bring about impaired functioning. Other conditions which cause death less frequently, but which also impair functioning, are arthritis and other orthopedic conditions, high blood pressure, diabetes, chronic brain syndrome, and sense organ problems. Unlike people with short-term illness, the elderly are more likely to suffer from two or more conditions simultaneously. In addition, the chronically ill face constant risks such as physical deterioration and psychological and social problems, including economic dependency, decreased social interaction, geographic confinement, lack of mental stimulation, and the psychological stresses of disability, pain, and impending death (Katz et al. 1975).

As reported in *Forward Plan for Health, 1978–82* (U.S. DHEW 1976a), a number of serious problems and deficiencies have been uncovered in recent assessments of the status of long-term care from a national perspective. One of these problems is inadequate planning for the development and utilization of essential services and resources. Long-term care consumes a larger portion of national health expenditures than was anticipated. For example, in 1975, nursing expenditures amounted to $9 billion, which was a $1.5 billion increase over 1974. The bulk of these expenditures was derived from the Medicare and Medicaid programs, neither of which was designed to deal with long-term care.

Other problems and deficiencies in long-term care identified in the *Forward Plan* include: changes in the traditional role of the family and the community in responding to the needs of their members; too little attention given to the role of preventive efforts in delaying and/or eliminating the onset of chronic disabling conditions, degeneration, and dependency; lack of structured health education activities to encourage adoption of a basic life style that promotes health maintenance rather than physical dependence; and deficiencies in the administrative, managerial, and organizational arrangements for providing long-term care.

Of the 5 to 10 million adults who might have needed some form of long-term care in 1975, it can be estimated that from 1.9 to 2.7 million received assistance from formal programs. Of these, 1.6 million are in institutions and 75,000 to 635,000 are in other types of sheltered living arrangements. Up to 500,000 people are served by home health agencies under Medicare and Mecicaid and also receive help from relatives. It is assumed that noninstitutionalized disabled persons living with others are receiving informal or basic care from their families. An estimated 800,000 to 1.4 million disabled may receive no form of long-term care (U.S. Congress 1977).

A study by Shanas and associates (1968) addressed various social phenomena among older persons in three industrial societies: Denmark, Great Britain, and the United States. Structured interviews were conducted with approximately 2,500 persons in each country who were age sixty-five and over and were living in private households. The study examined the level of physical functioning of older people, how they used community services, their relationships with family and friends, and their economic position. In her study, Shanas used the condition of those who were institutionalized as an indicator of the general level of physical functioning of older people in these countries. She found that more than half of those in institutions in the United States and Great Britain were in hospitals or nursing homes and, with some exceptions, can be assumed to be either bedfast or in need of nursing care. In Denmark, one third of those in institutions were believed to be non-ambulatory and bedfast. In each of the three countries, it was found that the proportion of older people who were either bedfast or house-bound but had managed to remain living at home was greater than the proportion of older people in each country residing in institutions.

Shanas used an index of incapacity to measure the functioning of elderly people. Her index was similar to the index of Independence in Activities of Daily Living (ADL) first developed by Katz and his associates, (1963) and used in this Chronic Disease Module study. The Shanas study provided several relevant findings: younger persons had fewer incapacities than older persons; persons aged sixty-five to sixty-nine in all three countries functioned quite well as measured by the index of incapacity; the percentage of persons who experience difficulty with common physical tasks rises with each advance in age.

The presence of chronic conditions was cited in *Long-Term Care for the Elderly and Disabled* (U.S. Congress 1977) as one indicator of need for long-term care, but not the only determinant of need. The need for assistance in activities of daily living such as eating, bathing, and toileting was found to be a better gauge. That there is a relatively higher rate of functional disability among the elderly is well established. Between 11.8% and 16.8% of the population over sixty-five is estimated to be functionally disabled. Based on the incidence of functional disability, the total potential demand for long-term care is estimated to increase between 5.5 and 9.9 million persons in 1975 to between 6.3 and 11.1 million in 1980 and to between 7.4 and 12.5 million in 1985.

The Forward Plan for Health, 1977–81 (U.S. DHEW 1975b) reported that in 1972 an estimated 6.5 million persons or 3.2% of the civilian, noninstitutionalized population were hampered by one or more chronic conditions. About 1.8 million of these persons were confined to the house, of which one-fourth were confined to bed. Another 2.1 million needed help in movement, either from a special device or another person. Furthur, the probability of living in institutions after age sixty-five appears to depend on the combined influence of age, marital status, race, and sex. In 1975 over 80% of the males and almost 60% of the females over sixty-five years of age were living outside of institutions with a spouse, relatives, or someone else.

An area of great concern at present is the continued health maintenance of the chronically ill, disabled, or aged patient. Greater continuity in care is the issue; the goal is to further autonomous behavior and to shift the emphasis of health care from institutions to home health care. A number of studies reported in the literature during the last decade have contributed a greater understanding of the continuing health care needs of the chronically ill aged. Jones (1974) found that 84% of a sample of chronically ill ambulatory patients had health care problems—66% had three or more health care problems of varying types. Patients most frequently needed help with medication, nutritional requirements, physical care such as exercise and skin care, and in emotional/behavioral areas. Jones found a need for improvement in the care functions of assessment, monitoring of physical and psychosocial status, education and support of the patient and family in long-term management of a treatment regimen within the context of activities of daily living, and facilitation of the use of existing family and community resources.

Forrester and Hill (1975) believed that the needs of the chronically ill for ambulatory services can be met if our health care delivery system can reallocate present resources and, where feasible, utilize trained health care assistants to extend the capacity of the primary care physician and specialist. To manage home care given by a health assistant most efficiently, they suggested an enrollment procedure for purposes of screening, education of the patient about health assistant care, and establishment of the health assistant's identity within the clinical setting. Following these steps, it was suggested that an initial health assessment should be performed, a problem list developed, and subsequent plans for adequate follow-up made with as much of the care as possible being administered by the health assistant.

Sidney Katz and his associates (1972, 1970, 1969, 1968, 1967) have provided long-term epidemiologic studies of chronic illness, experimental studies of health services, methodological studies involving measurement and assessment of physical, psychological, and social function, and studies of the effectiveness of multidiciplinary health care and home care.

In Cleveland, Ohio, Katz and his associates (1968) also conducted a controlled study of comprehensive outpatient care of rheumatoid arthritis patients with coordinated care provided by staff members of the University Hospitals and the Visiting Nurse Association. They found that continued outpatient treatment, when compared to the usual form of care, yielded positive results—the clinical manifestations of the disease itself showed fewer deteriorations and more improvements; there were more improvements and fewer deteriorations in economic dependence and fewer regressions in daily activities and performance.

HOME CARE FOR THE CHRONICALLY ILL

Providers concerned with care for the chronically ill elderly have maintained for at least a generation that whenever possible the patient's own home should be utilized for long-term care rather than the often depersonalized institutional setting. It is a recognized fact that much of the care currently provided in institutional settings could be as effectively and moré economically provided in the home.

Somers and Moore (1976) pointed out that although there is agreement on potential cost savings as well as a strong preference of most of the elderly and chronically ill to remain in their own homes, health care in the United States remains heavily institution-oriented. A primary explanation is the reimbursement policies of federal and state programs. All home health programs account for less than 1% of Medicare expenditures and an estimated 4% of federal-state expenditures under Medicaid. Other factors that militate against the growth of care in the home are: the overwhelming priority that physicians and most health care professionals give to care for acute illness rather than to prevention and management of chronic illness; the fear among third party payors that there will be a high incidence of abuse because noninstitutional care is more difficult to monitor; the typically small urban apartment; and the smaller number of children to share the burden of providing care for aged and chronically ill parents.

Forward Plan for Health, 1978–82 (U.S. DHEW, 1976a) described plans for experiments and demonstrations to test the feasibility of homemaker, day care, and day hospitalization services under authority of Section 222 of P.L. 92–603. One of the objectives in this federal document is based on indications that home health care programs are a cost-effective and humane ingredient in the continuum of care, and release valuable institutional resources to treat patients with more complex health care requirements. Greater utilization of home health services will be promoted by resolving the problems of reimbursement for these services by Medicare and Medicaid.

The Division of Nursing, Health Resources Administration, surveyed a variety of agencies, including local health departments, visiting nurse associations, hospital- and institution-based home care units, community or neighborhood health centers, and other types of local organizations that deliver care to the home in an effort to delineate the activities of home care service. As reported in *The Nation's Use of Health Resources* (U.S. DHEW 1976b), a total of 179,397,400 visits were made during a one-year period. Of these, 32,675,300 were made by local health agencies, and

918,300 by hospital-administered programs. The remainder represents direct or telephone contacts by physicians.

The role of hospitals in the delivery of home care services was studied by the American Hospital Association and also reported in *The Nation's Use of Health Resources*. A 1972 survey showed that more than 918,000 home care visits were provided by 225 hospital-administered programs in 1971,

Home care programs in this country vary widely in their size, scope, and base of operations. The focus of most home care programs, however, is the chronically ill patient. Some home care programs are intended to provide a substitute for in-hospital treatment (Gerson and Berry 1976; Queen 1976). Others emphasize health maintenance and the values of home care as an alternative to long-term institutionalization (Brickner et al. 1976 Bryant et al. 1974; Burch 1975; Katz et al. 1972; Kovar 1977).

Brickner et al. (1976) described the development of the Chelsea Village Program based at St. Vincent's Hospital, Manhattan. It was begun in response to the needs of the elderly for medical attention through outreach services in their homes. The study involved 245 patients in a New York City program for the homebound aged. It was reported that after two years 23 patients had improved to the extent that they were no longer homebound, 116 remained stabilized under the program's continuing care, and 40 patients were institutionalized in either a hospital or nursing home. Brickner and his associates estimated that 85 of the patients would have required institutional care and 25 of the patients would have died if they had not participated in the program.

A home health services survey conducted by Van Dyke and Brown (1972) had the following objectives: (1) to describe the care received by patients of organized home health agencies in the New York Metropolitan Area; (2) to relate the services given to the needs of the patients; and (3) to determine the position of home health services in the total picture of health care delivery. The results reinforced the tenet that home health care was both a desirable and appropriate alternative to institutionalization. The services offered, however, were judged as needing improvement in two-thirds of the sample studied.

A randomized controlled study by Gerson and Hughes (1976) measured the efficacy of the early transfer of hospital in-patients to home care. Patients undergoing one of five surgical procedures were used in the study, which measured their rates of return to normal role functions in work, leisure, and household roles. The conclusion was that after three weeks following discharge from either a home care program or a hospital, there were no significant differences in rates of return to work or leisure between a control group who remained in the hospital for the usual length of time and a group of patients who were transferred to a home care regimen. For four out of five categories of household tasks, home care patients performed a greater percentage of normal tasks; in two of these categories the difference was significant.

From their study of alternative living arrangements for the elderly in Louisville, Kentucky, Bradshaw et al. (1976) formulated several suggestions to improve foster home care for the aged and minimally impaired. Among the considerations suggested were: (1) have both nursing and social services available for assistance to the operators of the program; (2) make support services available so that the elderly can engage in community groups appropriate to their interests; (3) evaluate the elderly to be placed in the program for more serious problems that perhaps should be handled elsewhere (e.g., alcoholism); and (4) provide enough economic backing to insure a consistent high quality of home health care to the residents involved in the program.

One of the more important factors involved in the evaluation of the effectiveness of a home health care program is the cost of such programs as compared to the cost of the traditional hospital recuperation stay.

If a program is said to be "cost-effective," this indicates that it can accomplish a stated goal more cheaply than can an alternative program. A study measuring the cost-effectiveness of home health care was done by LaVor and Callender (1976). The major problem that they encountered in comparing home care with institutional care was in developing techniques so that the costs could be measured and expressed in equivalent terms. Costs for institutional care are generally available only as costs per day, which includes room, board, and personal care. Home care costs are often measured only in "per item of service" terms, which reflect only health services.

The conclusions reached by these authors concerning the methods that must be developed before a sound cost-effectiveness analysis can be undertaken were: (1) cost accounting systems must be standardized among hospitals, nursing homes, and home health agencies; (2) data must be obtained for all patients on a case basis, a per diem basis, and a diagnostic basis regardless of the care modality; (3) cost elements must be listed and categorized on equivalent bases; (4) costs must be related to the level of care given to permit adequate comparison between modalities; (5) patients with comparable characteristics must be selected at data sources for each modality (i.e., comparability of diagnosis, impairment levels, intensity of illness, and economic and social resources available); and (6) in the noninstitutional setting, other public costs such as the amount of income support need to be accounted for. One further factor to be considered is the impact upon cost calculations of the key health, demographic, social, and economic characteristics of the population served. Therefore, "home care for whom" and "home care for what purpose" are salient questions.

In studies of the cost-effectiveness of home care, services have been categorized as being one of two types. The most common type is acute or intensive, where home care is evaluated as an alternative to hospital care or to some part of the normal hospital stay. The second type is intermediate care, which requires somewhat less skilled or frequent visits with more basic care than acute care. The type of care category must be examined in relation to equivalent levels of institutional care to achieve a fair evaluation. The overall cost-effectiveness study must take a long range view and consider the impact of home care on the individual, on the health care system, and on the state and federal governments. In the immediate future, the expansion of home care programs could lead to an increase in program expenditures for all types of care rather than a substitution of home care for other types of care. Time is needed to counteract present trends toward the increased cost of and utilization of hospitals and nursing homes. A need will still remain for these institutions, but it is hoped that hospital stays can be shortened and entry into institutions can be prevented where possible by the implementation of home care programs.

The goal of such programs is to develop an alternative in health care that has higher quality outcomes than those presently offered, and that will lead to better quality living for the patients involved. LaVor and Callender (1976) noted that further research is needed on their home care program to thoroughly evaluate the impact it has upon the elderly. Some questions still to be answered are: Does it impede the process of deterioration in the health of the elderly? Does it enhance the social and psychological well-being of the subscribers? Does it provide a more economical alternative to higher levels of health care?

In measuring the impact of home care services on the hospital utilization patterns of 100,000 members of the Kaiser Foundation Health Plan, the Kaiser Study (Hurtado 1969) demonstrated that home care alone did not significantly reduce the cost of acute care for their membership, but that it did contribute to the overall well-being of a significant number of patients. The direction of the home care services offered in this study was changed from a traditional emphasis on nursing care only to an emphasis on providing the services of a nurse, social worker, and physical therapist as well as other support personnel. At the end of the project, the home care agency staff included a director, nursing supervisor, social work supervisor, physical therapy supervisor, three public health nurses, one registered nurse, one licensed practical nurse, and eight home health aides. It is interesting to note that the home health aides performed 48% of all procedures, and the professionals reported that the aides provided effective field service.

In a controlled study that served as a basis for the model of home care which is the subject of this book, Katz et al. (1972), measured the effects of home nursing care on patients discharged from a chronic disease rehabilitation hospital. As noted in the previous chapter, this study contributed specific information about the outcomes of the home service program.

A related one-year study by Nielsen et al. (1972) explored the effect of organized home aide service on patients discharged from a geriatric rehabilitation hospital and on the older members of their households. They found that they could make no definitive statements on survival rates in comparing service and control groups. They found, however, that there was greater contentment and less institutionalization among the service participant group.

A major task or objective of the model of home care services discussed in this book is to enable health service organizations to carry out their functions in a less fragmented manner and to facilitate availability, sensitivity, and continuity of care. One of the requirements for the development of the type of home care provided was the belief that the management of chronic illness must be individualized according to the nature and degree of illness, associated problems, and environmental circumstances (Commission on Chronic Illness 1957).

NEW HEALTH CARE MANPOWER

One of the major gaps in the provision of services to the chronically ill and aged is the lack of professional manpower with specialized training in long-term care. In general, the training of health care personnel has not engendered a sensitivity to the full range of complex medical, nursing, and social needs of long-term patients. As noted in *Forward Plan for Health, 1978–82* (U.S. DHEW 1976a), federal manpower policy has emphasized programs to increase the total number of health personnel. The critical manpower issue, however, is not one of absolute numbers but one of directing the growing manpower resources into areas of recognized need.

In the last decade many new types of health manpower have emerged (Gartner 1973; Glaser 1972; Kissick 1968; Perry 1969.) Various levels of specialized and generalized health professionals have been trained, including health associates and pediatric nurse practitioners (Silver, Ford, and Day 1968), anesthesia assistants, and physician assistants (Stead 1967). In addition, new categories of less trained but highly skilled health workers who work with health professionals have been developed, e.g., the family health worker of the Montefiore Neighborhood Medical Care Demonstration (Wise et al. 1968), the health aide of the Yale Family Health Care Project (Beloff and Willett 1968), and the community health aide of the Contra Costa Project in California (Luckham and Swift 1969). The basic impact of these new health workers on health services to the chronically ill in their homes has yet to be determined.

Mark (1974) noted that the use of new manpower types has strong advocates, but that many providers of health care are reluctant to burden themselves with collection of economic and operational data. If services rendered by allied health manpower are to be made generally reimbursable, it seems evident that such information would be required by third parties.

The use of new health manpower by the Kaiser Foundation was found to be effective in achieving better coordination of patient care (Hurtado 1969). The home health aides participated in an eight-week program which originally reflected a heavy nursing influence, but later was modified to provide more emphasis on rehabilitation and social service. The aides were trained and supervised by the health professionals (nurse, social worker, occupational therapist, and physical therapist) whose services they were to assume. The study reported that this led to greater communication among the professionals as well as between the professionals and the aides.

Morrow (1973) described a program developed in conjunction with a junior college for the training of health assistants to help bridge the gap between professional health personnel and the community, especially among minority ethnic groups. The advantages of this program seem to lie in the fact that health assistants were able to assume responsibility for many of the routine tasks previously performed by more highly trained personnel.

The services offered in our study, as described in Chapter 5, utilized health assistants as part of a medical unit within the health service system. The health assistants were supported in their role by the more professionally prepared medical specialists of the team and developed their own norms of operation under the supervison of the professionals in accordance with the particular demands placed on them.

INTERDISCIPLINARY TEAM CARE

Concurrent with the development of new health manpower is the use of interdisciplinary teams for the delivery of comprehensive, continuing, and coordinated health services. The concept of team care has an especially important place in today's thinking about care of patients with long-term illness (Katz, Halstead, and Wierenga 1975).

The literature about health care delivery by interdisciplinary teams is prolific, but the absence of common concepts and perspectives makes difficult the effective communication that could lead to the pursuit of common objectives and solving of common problems. There is general agreement among authors that an interdisciplinary team approach is a highly acceptable way of providing care to chronically ill patients, but the degree to which or manner in which it enhances patient care have not been the subject of any controlled or comparative studies.

Abdellah (1970) studied the training and development of workers for the health care team, and defined it as a group of health professionals trained at various levels and often at different institutions working together to provide health care. She stated that the impetus for the development of new models of health care delivery staffing is the scarcity of highly trained personnel and the need to have less complex functions performed by persons with less training. The health care team can therefore serve to increase the availability of health services.

The issues in the area of optimum organization facing primary care teams in most health systems are complex, involving both the patient care system and the health delivery system (Beckhard 1972). The key issue would seem to be the preparation of individuals during their educational training to work as team members. Barriers to the effective functioning of health teams have been analyzed by Wise et al. (1974). Some of the problems identified were issues of power and leadership, team members' assumption of family surrogate roles, and communication issues. The background and training of team members, and their level of preparation for the roles they are expected to assume, helps or hinders their

effective functioning on the team. In an attempt to meet these training needs at Martin Luther King Neighborhood Health Center,
specialists in organization development studied the top administration as well as the individual teams. Teams were given a variety of
data about their mode of functioning, and the administration was
restructured to give more authority to the health teams and to
provide them with more effective back-up services.

The internal dynamics involved when individuals attempt to
function as a group was the focus of a study by Rubin and Beckhard
(1972). The authors outlined five characteristics that are key to
group functioning: (1) goals or mission, (2) internal and external
role expectations, (3) decision-making, (4) communication patterns and leadership, and (5) norms.

Certain aspects of health care teams and their effectiveness have
been the subject of controlled studies. Bakst and Marna (1955)
described a home care program for cardiac patients that included
many of the same elements in its research design as are employed
in the present study: random assignment of patients into two groups,
definition of characteristics by which patients were screened for in-
clusion in the study, prospective collection of data, selection of a
population so that treatment can be introduced to one group without altering the methods of receiving care to the other group, and
the collection of information on such items as number of visits, the
characteristics of members of the team, cost factors, and outcome
data on institutionalizations, morbidity, and mortality.

A study by Nash (1974) placed emphasis on the importance of
physician input relative to the referral procedure. Other home care
studies using the team approach demonstrated the utilization of
allied health professionals in extending the capacity of the physician
and nurse. (Forrester and Hill 1975; How 1973; Hurtado 1969;
Nielsen et al. 1972.)

McQue and Chughtai (1975) presented a model by which the
medical and social needs of the elderly were met in their home
through the parallel work of two teams of professional personnel
with well-defined roles whose work was coordinated by a physician.
One problem with this study was that team conferences, which are
seen as essential to the delivery of comprehensive coordinated care,
were not used. The use of professionals to render home health care

would also seem to prevent the lowering of the cost of home health care to a level which can be sustained by society.

The number of controlled studies describing the impact specific program of services for the care of the chronically ill elderly in their homes is very limited. The need for research programs and mechanisms for translating research findings so that they can be used by administrators of health service programs, practitioners, families, and communities is apparent.

REFERENCES

Abdellah, F. G. 1970. Training and development of workers for the health care team. *AORN Journal* 11:86–91.

Bakst, H. J., and Marna, E. F. 1955. Experience with home care for cardiac patients. *AJPH* 45:444–450.

Beckhard, R. 1972. Organizational issues in the team delivery of comprehensive health care. *Milbank Memorial Fund Quarterly* 50:287–315.

Beloff, J. S., and Willett, M. 1968. Yale studies in family health care Ill. The health care team. *JAMA* 205:663–669.

Bradshaw, B. R., Vonderhaar, W. P., Keeney, V. T., et al. 1976. Community-based residential care for the minimally impaired elderly: A survey analysis. *Journal of Amer. Geriatric Society* 24:423–429.

Brickner, P. W., Janeski, J. F., Rich, G., and Duque, S. T. 1976. Home maintenance for the homebound aged. *The Gerontologist* 16:25–29.

Bryant, N. H., Candland, L., and Loewenstein, R. 1974. Comparison of care and cost outcomes for stroke patients, with and without home care. *Stroke* 5:54–59.

Burch, G. E. 1975. A need for more care at home. *American Heart Journal* 89:402–403.

Commission on Chronic Illness. 1956. *Chronic Illness in the United States II: Care of the Long-Term Patient.* Cambridge: Harvard University Press.

Forrester, R. H., and Hill, C. L. 1975. Improving care of the chronically ill. *Hospitals* 49:57–62.

Gartner, A. 1973. Health systems and new careers. *Health Services Reports* 88:124–130.

Gerson, L. W., and Berry, A. F. E. 1976. Psycho-social effects of home care. Results of a randomized controlled trial. *International Journal of Epidemiology* 5:159–165.

Gerson, L. W., and Hughes, O. P. 1976. A comparative study of the economics of home care. *International Journal of Health Services* 6:543–555.

Glaser, R. J. 1972. Health care and education. In U.S. Department of Health, Education, and Welfare, *Technology and Health Care Systems in the 1980's*, Proceedings of a Conference, 1972, San Francisco, California.

How, N. M. 1973. A team caring for the elderly at home. *Journal of the Royal College of General Practitioners* 23:627–637.

Hurtado, A. V. 1969. Integration of home health and extended care facility services into a prepaid, comprehensive group practice plan. DHEW Contract #PH 110–196. June 28, 1967–September 1, 1969.

Jones, P. E. 1974. Nursing needs of ambulatory patients with chronic disease. *Canadian Journal of Public Health* 65:422–426.

Katz, S., Downs, T. D., Cash, H. R., and Grotz, R. C. 1970. Progress in development of the Index of ADL. *The Gerontologist* 10:20–30.

Katz, S., Ford, A. B., Downs, T. D., and Adams, M. 1969. Chronic disease classification in evaluation of medical care programs. *Medical Care* 7:139–143.

Katz, S., Ford, A. B., Downs, T. D., Adams, M., and Rusby, D. 1972. *Effects of Continued Care: A Study of Chronic Illness in the Home.* DHEW Publication No. (HSM) 73–3010. U.S. Government Printing Office, Washington, D.C.

Katz, S., Ford, A. B., Heiple, K. G., and Newill, V. A. 1964. Studies of illness in the aged: Recovery after fracture of the hip. *Journal of Gerontology* 19:285–293.

Katz, S., Ford, A. B., Moskowitz, R. W., Jackson, B. A., and Jaffe, N. W. 1963. Studies of illness in the aged: The Index of ADL: A standardized measure of biological and psychosocial function. *JAMA* 185:914–919.

Katz, S., Halstead, L., and Wierenga, M. 1975. A medical perspective. In Sherwood, S. (ed.) *Long-Term Care: A Handbook for Researchers, Planners, and Providers.* New York: Spectrum Publications, Inc.

Katz, S., Heiple, K. G., Downs, T. D., Ford, A. B., and Scott, C. P. 1967. Long-term course of 147 patients with fracture of the hip. *Surgery, Gynecology and Obstetrics* 124:1219–1230.

Katz, S., Vignos, P. J., Jr., Moskowitz, R. W., Thompson, H. M., and Svec, K. 1968. Comprehensive outpatient care in rheumatoid arthritis, a controlled study. *JAMA* 206:1249–1254.

Kissick, W. L. 1968. Health manpower in transition. *Milbank Memorial Fund Quarterly* 46:53–90.

Kovar, M. G. 1977. Health of the elderly and use of health services. *Public Health Reports* 92:9–19.

LaVor, J. L., and Callender, M. 1976. Home health cost effectiveness: What are we measuring? *Medical Care* 14:866–872.

Luckham, J., and Swift, D. 1969. Community health aides in the ghetto: The Contra Costa Project. *Medical Care* 7:332–339.

Mark, R. 1974. Brandeis Conference on Paramedical Personnel. *Health Services Research* 9:159–162.

McQue, J. G., and Chughtai, M. A. 1975. The importance of team work in geriatric care. *Nursing Times* 71:140–142.

Morrow, R. C. 1973. The training of health assistants. *Health Services Reports* 88:588–590.

Nash, D. T. 1974. Making use of home care services. *Geriatrics* 29:140–145.

Nielson, M., Beggs, H., and Blenkner, M. 1972. Older persons after hospitalization: A controlled study of home health aide services. *AJPH* 62:1094–1101.

Perry, J. W. 1969. Career mobility in allied health education. *JAMA* 210:107–120.

Queen, J. E. 1976. The Blue Cross and Blue Shield Coordinated Home Care Program. *Maryland State Medical Journal* 25:42–43.

Rubin, I., and Beckhard, R. 1972. Factors influencing the effectiveness of the health team. *Milbank Memorial Fund Quarterly* 50:317–335.

Shanas, E., Townsend, P., Wedderburn, D., Friis, H., Milhøj, P., and
Stenhouwer, J. 1968. *Old People in Three Industrial Societies.* New York:
Atherton Press.
Silver, H. K., Ford, L., and Day, L. 1968. The pediatric nurse practitioner
program. *JAMA* 204:298–302.
Somers, A. R., and Moore, F. M. 1976. Homemaker services—essential
option for the elderly. *Public Health Reports* 91:354–359.
Stead, E. A. 1967. The Duke Plan for physician's assistants. *Medical Times*
95:40–48.
U.S. Congress. Congressional Budget Office. 1977. *Long-Term Care for the
Elderly and Disabled.* Budget Issue Paper. Y10.12:E1.2. U.S. Govern-
ment Printing Office, Washington, D.C.
U.S. Department of Health, Education, and Welfare. 1975. Division of
Nursing, Health Resources Assoc. Survey. In Bureau of Health Manpower
Surveys of Public Health Nursing 1968–1972. DHEW Publication No.
(HRA) 76–8. U.S. Government Printing Office, Washington, D.C.
U.S. Department of Health, Education, and Welfare. 1975b. *Forward Plan
for Health FY1977–81.* DHEW Publication No. (OS) 76–50024. U.S.
Government Printing Office, Washington, D.C.
U.S. Department of Health, Education, and Welfare. 1976a. *Forward Plan
for Health FY1978–82.* DHEW Publication No. (OS) 76–50046. U.S.
Government Printing Office, Washington, D.C.
U.S. Department of Health, Education, and Welfare. 1976b. *The Nation's
Use of Health Resources.* DHEW Publication No. (HRA) 77–1240. U.S.
Government Printing Office, Washington, D.C.
Van Dyke, F., and Brown, V. 1972. Organized home care: an alternative
to institutions. *Inquiry* 9:3–16.
Wise, H. B., Torrey, E. F., McDade, A., Perry, G., and Bograd, H. 1968.
The family health worker. *AJPH* 58:1828–1838.
Wise, H. B., et al. 1974. *Making Health Teams Work.* Ballinger Publishing
Company.

Chapter 3

RESEARCH PLAN
AND METHODS

Carole Bettinghaus
Sidney Katz
Sister Mary Honora Kroger

Simply stated, the design of our experiment involved random assignment of people to treatment and control groups. Observations were then made to determine whether the results in one group were better than in the other group. With the aid of appropriate statistical techniques, we made interpretations about the benefit or lack of benefit by the service program, as well as about differences in the use of health services and the charges for such services.

What appears to be a simple design, however, is complex; and the ideal experiment is not attainable in social experiments such as this. For example, the population from which the participants came is difficult to describe in terms that allow universal generalizations. The process of random assignment helped to avoid certain biases, but ethical considerations required that participants choose for themselves, in a nonrandom manner, how much service they would accept. Some, in fact, refused to accept service even after being referred to service. In the larger demonstration types of community experiments, external community forces may resist the experiments—as, for example, professional care providers who are concerned with possible encroachment on their spheres of influence, and administrators or directors of services who may find it difficult to incorporate investigative processes into their daily activities.

Complex service programs such as the one in this experiment are difficult to describe in their entirety. Although participants were assigned to service and control groups in a pure sense, they did not always receive clearly separate and different services. Control patients may have indirectly received certain elements of care that were reserved for the service group. If control and service patients came into contact with each other, they may have influenced each other; and if this so-called "contaminating influence" was large, service benefits could have been obscured.

It is also evident that reliable and meaningful measures are needed that are sensitive to changes in the health status of participants if we are to draw conclusions about whether the treatment group responded better than the control group. The mere proposal of a classification system does not establish its usefulness as a measure of effectiveness. A great deal of background research is needed. In the absence of established and tested measures, there is often a tendency to accumulate overly detailed information in the hope that success or failure will be revealed in the details. In this regard, it has been repeatedly observed that much effort in accumulating such information is found to have been wasted when the results are later reported. Furthermore, the multidisciplinary (i.e., physical, psychological, social, and economic) aspects of chronic illness make it desirable to use multidisciplinary measures of effectiveness; and the available number is limited. Investigators are thus faced with the difficult choice of being selective or designing impractically cumbersome, detailed studies.

These and many other issues faced us as we planned and conducted this study. Basically, we recognized that the ideal conditions of a textbook experiment could not be achieved. Our responsibility was to approach the optimal study requirements as best we could and, then, to make cautious interpretations that reflected both the findings and the constraints of circumstances in which the study was carried out.

RESEARCH DESIGN

The basic plan of the study was to use the experimental method to the extent possible in this type of community-focused social research. Accordingly, we randomly assigned disabled persons for whom health services were judged appropriate to treatment and control groups. The experimental treatment consisted of services delivered in the home by members of a health care team called the Chronic Disease Module. The team included a half-time nurse or social worker, a part-time physician, and two full-time health assistants who were specifically trained to deliver care in the person's home. Persons in the control group received only the usual health support services offered within the community.

We planned to study the effects of service for one year because (1) a prolonged period of care was needed by the chronically disabled people who would be served, (2) the most measurable improvement for such patients would occur during the first year after treatment began, and (3) the expected mortality would result in a large decrease in sample size during the first year (Katz et al. 1966, 1967, 1972). Each participant was to be interviewed three times during a one-year period: at entry into the study, six months after entry, and twelve months after entry. The study design is diagrammed in Figure 3.1. Using this design, we studied the effects of the services by comparing results in the treatment group (i.e., "those referred to module service") and the control group (i.e., "those not referred to module service").

Since the persons in the study were of many different types, they were assigned randomly to treatment and control groups by a stratification process—that is, from smaller groups of similar age and sex. We also aimed to develop a sample size as large as available resources and time would allow, thereby permitting analysis of results in subgroups that included similar types of people.

Figure 3.1,

Plan of the Study

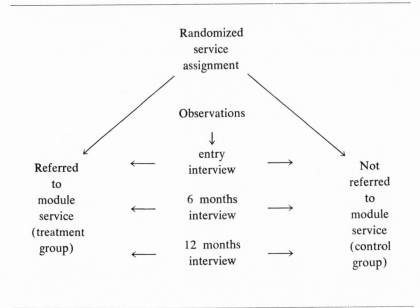

SELECTION AND ASSIGNMENT OF PATIENTS

Participants entered the study from five different communities in Michigan between August 1973 and June 1975. In order to identify those who could use module home services, we screened all persons who were either patients in selected ambulatory care facilities or who were about to be discharged from selected hospitals. The following criteria were used to define the eligibility of people for the study: (1) forty-five years of age or older, (2) discharged to, or living in, a noninstitutional setting within geographic access to the module service unit, (3) in need of assistance for at least three months with regard to either bathing, dressing, walking, cardiopulmonary conditions, or arthritis, and (4) not in need of either skilled nursing services, twenty-four-hour-a-day supervision, or kidney dialysis. Included as noninstitutional settings were the persons' own homes, the homes of relatives or friends, hotel residences, and state licensed foster homes. The screening questionnaire is presented in Appendix A. Selection criteria were designed to exclude people who were selfsufficient and unlikely to require home services, as well as those who were extremely disabled and likely to require institutional services.

After eligibility was determined, we assigned participants to a service group or to a control group, using a random process and stratifying on the basis of age and sex. We obtained the consent of all who participated. Table 3.1 compares the distribution by age and sex of people who were assigned to the study groups.

Table 3.1

Comparison of Number of Men and Woman in the
Assigned Study Groups By Age

	Referred to Module Service (Treatment Group)	*Not Referred to Module Service (Control Group)*
Men	177	175
45–61 years	55	56
62–74 years	78	75
75 yrs. plus	44	44
Women	261	261
45–61 years	73	81
62–74 years	102	93
75 yrs. plus	86	87
TOTAL	438	436

INFORMATION COLLECTED FOR THE STUDY

Information was collected that would allow description of the participants, comparison of those who accepted module services with those who did not, and evaluation of the response of those who were served. We also used the information to describe the use of services and to check the comparability of participants in the treatment and control groups. Additional information was collected for cost studies, to describe module services, to describe the community settings in which services were offered, and to describe the organization and function of the module team. Figure 3.2 presents a list of the measures that were used. Sources identified in the figure give details about the background and procedures concerning each measure. The evaluation schedule and forms for obtaining information are in Appendix B.

At the time of entry into the study, we evaluated each participant in terms of age, sex, race, marital status, rural or urban location, education, occupation, social position, type of residence, household composition, and residence of the person who gave the participant personal care. We also assessed the participant's physical, psychological, social, and economic functioning. We identified the diagnosis that led to the most recent hospital admission, using the International Code of Diseases, Adapted for Hospitals (H-ICDA) (Commission on Professional and Hospital Activities 1968). If a hospitalization did not precede entry into the study, we identified the diagnosis that was associated with the patient's major disability.

During the six-month and twelve-month interviews, we obtained additional information about the family's income, source of payment for health care, and recent events of social deprivation in terms of personal loss and change in social role. We reviewed current status with regard to type of residence, household composition, and residence of the individual who gave personal care. At six and twelve months, we also reevaluated physical, psychological, social, and economic functioning. Finally, we recorded information about institutionalization, module services that we received, other health services that were received, and the charges for the latter.

Many of the measures used in the study had been successfully used in *Effects of Continued Care* (Katz et al. 1972). The demonstrated utility of the measures in that study, and the desire to compare findings between the two studies, contributed to the decision to apply them in this study as well.

Measures of function served both to describe the participants at entry and to measure their responses at later times. Measures of activities of daily living, walking, and mobility had been developed and applied by the authors during more than seventeen years. One of these, the Index of Independence in Activities of Daily Living, is a sociobiologic measure that ranks people according to their level

Figure 3.2

Measures in the Study

Measures to Characterize Participants	Measures That Evaluate the Effects of Module Service
Age	Activities of Daily Living (Katz et al. 1976)
Sex	Walking (Katz et al. 1964)
Race	Mobility (Jones et al. 1973)
Diagnosis (H-ICDA) (Commission on Professional and Hospital Activities 1968)	Bed Disability (U.S. Dept. of Health, Education, and Welfare 1976)
Activities of Daily Living (Katz et al. 1976)	Death
Walking (Katz et al. 1964)	Economic Dependence (Katz et al. 1972)
Bed Disability (U.S. Dept. of Health, Education, and Welfare 1976)	Satisfaction/Contentment (Bloom & Blenkner 1970)
Marital Status	Orientation (MSQ) (Kahn et al. 1960)
Education	Observation and Clear Thinking (Raven 1962)
Occupation	Social Role Activities (adapted from Spitzer et al. 1971)
Social Position (Hollingshead Two-Factor Index) (Hollingshead 1957)	Institutionalization
Family Income	in hospitals
Source of Payment for Health Care	in long-term care facilities
Economic Dependence (Katz et al. 1972)	Duration of Noninstitutional Living
Rural or Urban Location	Health Services Received
Type of Residence	Charges for Health Care
Household Composition	
Residence of Person Who Gives Personal Care	
Satisfaction/Contentment (Bloom & Blenkner 1970)	
Orientation (MSQ) (Kahn et al. 1960)	
Observation and Clear Thinking (Raven 1962)	
Recent Personal Loss or Role Change (Shanas et al. 1968)	
Social Role Activities (adapted from Spitzer et al. 1971)	
Intensity of Module Care	

* Citations in parentheses can be located in the reference list at the end of the chapter.

of dependence in six basic functions, namely, bathing, dressing, going to toilet, transferring, continence, and feeding (Katz and Akpom, 1976; Staff of Benjamin Rose Hospital 1959). In a single summary grade, the index reflects the adequacy of a person's organized neurological and locomotor behavior. A particularly useful characteristic of this measure is the hierarchical relationship among the activities contained in the scale. Its basic nature has been supported by the observation that the order in which independent functions are regained parallels the functional development of children. The usefulness of the measure has been demonstrated in numerous epidemiologic studies, in surveys, and in experiments.

The basic function, walking, was evaluated according to the following five-grade scale: walking by self, walking with mechanical assistance, walking with personal assistance, walking with mechanical and personal assistance, and not walking at all (Katz et al. 1964). We also evaulated the person's mobility, that is, the extent of the person's movement within his environment. As described in Jones's classification system, mobility was ranked as: going out of the house or institution without help, going out with mechanical aid (no personal assistance), going out with personal help only, going out with personal help and the aid of special devices, or confined indoors (Jones et al. 1973). We classified the amount of bed disability of each participant using definitions of the National Health Survey (U.S. DHEW 1976). When a study participant died, we recorded the date of death.

We believed that social factors would influence the acceptance of module care and the response to such care; thus we collected the identifying and sociodemographic information listed in Figure 3.2. We used one of the standard identifying and sociodemographic measures, Hollingshead's Two-Factor Index, which is based on education and occupation of the head of the household (Hollingshead 1957). We also used a measure of economic dependence which had been developed and used in related studies of a similar group of patients (Katz et al. 1972; Staff of Benjamin Rose Hospital 1961).

As a measure of social role activities, we inquired about the relative number of role activities that each participant had with spouse, family members and friends, and at work, adapted from a set of roles used by Spitzer (Spitzer et al. 1971). We also asked about any recent personal loss or change in role (Shanas et al. 1968). In particular, we asked about persons who moved away or died and about discontinuance of employment or homemaking. Participants then were classified according to the number of social deprivations that they had experienced.

We evaluated contentment or satisfaction by a short form of the Contentment Scale developed by Bloom and Blenkner (1970). To assess mental orientation, we used Kahn's Mental Status Questionnaire, a ten-item test that measures orientation with regard to time, place, and person (Kahn et al. 1958, 1960, 1961, 1962; Pollack et al. 1958). As a measure of observation and clear thinking, the Raven Coloured Progressive Matrices has been standardized for evaluation of elderly people and has been found to correlate well with the Wechsler Adult Intelligence Scale (Kidd 1962; Martin and Wiechers 1954; Raven 1962). The Raven test consists of sets of multiple choice problems arranged in order of increasing complexity. Each contains a graphic pattern from which a segment has been removed and six possible inserts from which the subject selects the matching insert. Since manual dexterity and the ability to speak are not necessary, it is very useful in testing aged and disabled people. It also covers a range of intellectual complexity that is appropriately discriminating of the capacities of old and disabled people.

INTERVIEWING AND DATA COLLECTION

Interviewers, recruited from each of the module service areas, had to be skilled in establishing rapport with study participants and their families (Kahn and Cannell 1963). They needed to be good listeners and had to record information accurately and objectively. An understanding of the aging process and chronic illness was required. Therefore, we hired interviewers who had previous public service experience, and carefully trained each for about forty hours. The training consisted of seminar discussions about chronic illness, aging, and principles of research interviewing. The background and purpose of each interview item was presented, and interviewers were taught how to record their observations. In role-playing sessions, the trainees practiced interviewing in both residential and institutional settings. Interviewers for the study were women between the ages of twenty-three and fifty-four. Most were married and college-educated. They were trained and supervised by persons with bachelor's degrees and with experience in health research interviewing.

In order to avoid biasing staff who delivered services in the home and staff who collected research information, we separated interviewers geographically and administratively from service personnel, and we prohibited interviewer involvement in service. Interviewers were not allowed access to information through which they would learn whether a participant was in the experimental or control group. We tried to have each participant interviewed by the same interviewer for all three interviews. This was done to provide continuity and to maintain rapport in subsequent contacts. In actual fact, about two-thirds of the participants had the same interviewer throughout the study.

The exact wording of questions and probes were specified in interview protocols, and data items on the interview schedule were precoded. In order to keep interviewer bias to a minimum, the interviewers avoided answering questions about care. Interviewers were instructed to make a first contact within one week of the assignment of participants to the study and to complete the first evaluation within two weeks. In difficult instances, interviewers were told to make at least three attempts to complete the interview. Delays were most often due to poor weather, poor road conditions in rural areas, or the participant's temporary residence outside of the area after discharge from a hospital.

Initial contact with a patient was always face-to-face and, in the case of hospitalized participants, was made before discharge whenever possible. Telephone contacts were made only when requested by the participant. Occasionally, follow-up evaluations were conducted during periods of hospitalization or institutionalization.

At the time of a first contact, the interviewer described her role and gave, or read, an explanatory brochure to the participant. Assurances of data confidentiality and individual anonymity were given. After the participant was fully informed about the research and had consented to be interviewed, the interviewer proceeded with the evaluation. At the end of each interview, the participant was told that there would be another interview in six months.

Most of the interviews were completed. Table 3.2, which summarizes the degree of completeness, indicates that a total of 2,622 interviews were theoretically possible. Of these, 10% were not conducted because the participants had died. Another 9% were not attempted because the data collection period had ended. Of the remaining 2,127 theoretically possible interviews, 89% were completed; 6% involved participants who had refused, could not be located, or had moved out of the area; and 5% were not attempted because there had not been complete prior interviews.

Although interviews were scheduled to be conducted immediately following entry into the study, and six and twelve months later, they were occasionally delayed because of such reasons as temporary acute illness of the participants, changes in address, and poor road or weather conditions. About two-thirds of the initial interviews were obtained within two weeks after entry, and about one-half of the six- and twelve-month interviews were obtained within two weeks before or after the date scheduled for the evaluation.

DATA PROCESSING AND ANALYSIS

All interview froms were edited by interview supervisors. Data were coded and checked for internal consistency by a central data controller and two coders. In addition, a 10% sample of the coding work was checked by the data controller, and a 10% sample of all coded interviews was coded by both coders. The two coders agreed in 19,665 out of 19,780 codes, representing better than 99% agreement in this reliability study.

Data were entered onto punch cards and run through a cleaning and verifying program. Only about 0.05% of 717,604 codes required correction of errors and inconsistencies. Data were stored in both a permanent computer disc file and a back-up magnetic tape file to guard against loss. Programs were developed to construct complex variables from the raw data, and a master program called the "data manager" controlled all output.

Table 3.2

Completion of Interviews

	Service Group			Control Group			Total Group		
	Initial	6-Month	12-Month	Initial	6-Month	12-Month	Initial	6-Month	12-Month
Completed interviews	409 (93.4%)	339 (77.4%)	190 (43.4%)	412 (94.5%)	346 (79.4%)	206 (47.2%)	821 (93.9%)	685 (78.4%)	396 (45.3%)
Interviews not completed or partly completed*	29 (6.6%)	46 (10.5%)	38 (8.7%)	24 (5.5%)	43 (9.9%)	45 (10.3%)	53 (6.1%)	89 (10.2%)	83 (9.5%)
Not eligible for interview:									
due to death	—	53 (12.1%)	85 (19.4%)	—	47 (10.8%)	73 (16.7%)	—	100 (11.4%)	158 (18.1%)
due to end of data collection period	—	—	125 (28.5%)	—	—	112 (25.7%)	—	—	237 (27.1%)
TOTALS	438	438	438	436	436	436	874	874	874

* These interviews were not completed or only partly completed because participants refused, could not be located, had moved out of the area, or had not completed interviews at the time of their prior interviews.

A major hypothesis in this study was that participants who received module service would maintain function better than those who did not receive such service—in other words, that those who were served would deteriorate less frequently. To test this hypothesis, we defined *effects* as *changes in function* from the time of entry into the study. This permitted us to treat each person as his/her own control and was conceptually equivalent to increasing the homogeneity of the study groups. As previously noted, completeness of the data was good. The study was designed to analyze the occurrence of death as one type of outcome and to exclude those who died in analyses of other outcomes. Users of the data can, thus, clearly understand the bases of our interpretations.

Using statistical tests, we checked the process of randomization, expecting that this process would balance out important extraneous factors (Chapter 6). We also used statistical tests to gain insight into possible explanations for non-acceptance of service by certain participants and to discover the effects of module service on outcome (Chapters 6 and 7). The chi-square test with continuity correction was applied and significance was set at the 95% level. The null hypothesis was rejected when p was ≤ 0.05. Regression analysis was used for the cost studies in Chapter 8, and significance levels were tested in analyses of variance using the F-test.

REFERENCES

Bloom, M. and Blenkner, M. 1970. Assessing functioning of older persons living in the community. *Gerontologist* 10:31–37.

Commission on Professional and Hospital Activities. 1968. *Hospital Adaptation of ICDA (H-ICDA)*. Published by Commission on Professional and Hospital Activities, Ann Arbor, Michigan.

Hollingshead, A. B. 1957. *Two Factor Index of Social Position*. New Haven: Hollingshead, pp. 1–11.

Jones, E. W., McNitt, B. J., and McKnight, E. M. 1973. *Patient Classification for Long-Term Care: User's Manual*. DHEW Publication No. (HRA) 74–3017. U.S. Government Printing Office, Washington, D.C.

Kahn, R. L. 1962. Measuring mental status in older patients. Paper presented at convention of American Psychological Association, August, 1962, St. Louis, Missouri.

Kahn, R. L., and Cannell, C. F. 1963. *The Dynamics of Interviewing*. New York: John Wiley & Sons, Inc., pp. 3–130, 203–232.

Kahn, R. L., Goldfarb, A. I., Pollack, M., and Gerber, I. E. 1958. The relationship of mental and physical status in institutionalized aged persons. Paper presented at 11th Annual Meeting of the Gerontological Society, November, 1958, Philadelphia, Pennsylvania.

Kahn, R. L., Goldfarb, A. I., Pollack, M., and Peck, A. 1960. Brief objective measures for the determination of mental status in the aged. *Am. J. Psychiatry* 117:326–328.

Kahn, R. L., Pollack, M., and Goldfarb, A. I. 1961. Factors related to individual differences in mental status of institutionalized aged. In Hoch, P. H., and Zubin, J., (eds.) *Psychopathology of Aging*. New York: Grune and Stratton.

Katz, S., and Akpom, C. A. 1976. A measure of primary sociobiological functions. *Int. J. Health Serv.* 6:493–508.

Katz, S., Ford, A. B., Chinn, A. B., and Newill, V. A. 1966. Prognosis after strokes. Part II, Long-term course of 159 patients, *Medicine* 45:236–246.

Katz, S., Ford, A. B., Downs, T. D., Adams, M., and Rusby, D. I. 1972. *Effects of Continued Care: A Study of Chronic Illness in the Home*. DHEW Publication No. (HSM) 73–3010. U.S. Government Printing Office, Washington, D.C.

Katz, S., Ford, A. B., Heiple, K. G., and Newill, V. A. 1964. Studies of illness in the aged: Recovery after fracture of the hip. *Journal of Gerontology* 19:285–293.

Katz, S., Ford, A. B., Moskowitz, R. W., Jackson, B. A., and Jaffe, M. W. 1963. Studies of illness in the aged: The Index of ADL. *JAMA* 185:914–919.

Katz, S., Heiple, K. G., Downs, T. D., Ford, A. B., and Scott, C. P. 1967. Long-term course of 147 patients with fracture of the hip. *Surgery, Gynecology and Obstetrics* 124:1219–1230.

Kidd, C. B. 1962. Criteria for admission of the elderly to geriatric and psychiatric units. *J. Ment. Sci.* 108:68–74.

Martin, A. S., and Wiechers, J. E. 1954. Raven's coloured progressive matrices and the Wechsler Intelligence Scale for children. *J. Consult. Psychol.* 18:143–144.

Pollack, M., Kahn, R. L., and Goldfarb, A. I. 1958. Factors related to individual differences in perception in institutionalized aged subjects. *Journal of Gerontology* 13:192–197.

Raven, J. C. 1962. *Coloured Progressive Matrices* (Sets A, Aв, B of revised order 1956). London: H. K. Lewis & Col, Ltd.

Shanas, E., Townsend, P., Wedderburn, D., Friis, H., Milhøj, P., and Stehouwer, J. 1968. *Old People in Three Industrial Societies*. New York: Atherton Press.

Spitzer, R. L., Gibbon, M., and Endicott, J. 1971. *Family Evaluation Form*. New York Department of Mental Hygiene data collection instrument.

Staff of the Benjamin Rose Hospital. 1959. Multidisciplinary studies of illness in aged persons: A new classification of functional status in activities of daily living. *J. Chron. Dis.* 9:55–62.

Staff of the Benjamin Rose Hospital. 1961. Multidisciplinary studies of illness in aged persons. V. A new classification of socio-economic functioning of the aged. *J. Chron. Dis.* 13:453–464.

U.S. Department of Health, Education, and Welfare. 1976. Persons injured and disability days. *Vital and Health Statistics Data from the National Health Survey*. DHEW Publication No. (HRA) 76–1532, Series 10 No. 105, U.S. Government Printing Office, Washington, D.C.

Chapter 4

MODULES AND
COMMUNITIES

Anne Cunningham
Carole Bettinghaus

The aim of the study was to establish module service in urban and
rural communities. In each community, we based the service module
in a host agency that had relationships with both primary services
and comprehensive referral services. We also wished to include a
variety of types of host agencies. As a basic requirement, administrators of host agencies had to indicate their explicit commitment to
strengthen the delivery of services to the chronically ill, as well as to
cooperate with the research requirement of the project.

Community organization activities extended throughout the duration of the project. Through such activities, host agencies were
identified and selected. Agency personnel and others in the community needed initial and continuing orientation about module
service and about the requirements of evaluation. Therefore orientation and continuing professional development activities for both
administrators and providers of service were conducted. We recruited
module staff and enlisted the cooperation of local community col-

leges to train health assistants. We established procedures to identify chronically ill people in the community who would be eligible for module service, and we established a process for their random referral to module service. Mechanisms for data collection were implemented, as were processes to coordinate data flow and monitor the quality of data. Much effort went into communicating the nature and purpose of the project to physicians, visiting nurses, and other providers of services in the community so that their cooperation would be maintained.

HOST AGENCIES, COMMUNITIES, AND MODULES

Service modules were established in five Michigan communities. Two were urban communities (populations of 220,000 to 420,000), and three were rural (populations of 20,000 to 45,000). After identifying the host agency in each community, the service module was integrated into the agency program. Modules were phased-in sequentially over a four-year period, and research elements were established concurrently. Figure 4.1, outlines the host agency, location, and team composition of the five modules.

Module A was established in a large city that already had two county agencies and three private agencies involved in home care. It was attached to a general hospital with 400 beds. As administrator of the module, the hospital's director assigned a deputy administrator who was also responsible for the ambulatory care programs of the hospital. This administrator maintained close contact with the service team and frequently attended case conferences. The physician member of the module team was the medical director of the family-oriented primary care clinic at the hospital. A master's level social worker was the other module professional. The module health assistants included one with partial prior training as a licensed practical nurse and one who had completed two years of college.

Module B was located in a rural community with a large percentage (11%) of people aged sixty-five years or older. The county had one of the lowest physician-population ratios in the state. There were three certified home health agencies, one of which served only cancer patients, in the county. Module B was attached to the

Figure 4.1

Host Agency and Community Setting Characteristics

Total Months of Module Service	*Type of Host Agency*	*Rural/Urban Location*	*Team Composition*
Module A 35	General acute care hospital	Urban	Physician, social worker, 2 health assistants
Module B 30	County health department (certified home care provider)	Rural	Physician, nurse, 2 health assistants
Module C 29	Ambulatory clinic	Rural	Physician, nurse, ** 2 health assistants
Module D 22	Ambulatory clinic	Urban	Physician, nurse, 2 health assistants
Module E 18	Clinic in housing unit for elderly*	Rural	Physician, nurse, 2 health assistants

* Subsequently located in a county medical care facility.
** Subsequently replaced by a bachelor's level social worker.

county health department and was administered by that department's administrator. Members of the module team included a local physician in private group practice, a master's level public health nurse, a health assistant who was also a licensed practical nurse, and a health assistant who had previously been a nurse's aide.

Module *C* was attached to a rural family health center that later became a health maintenance organization (HMO). The only other home care organization in the community was a hospital-based unit that offered skilled nursing services. The module was administered by the administrator of the health center. In addition to a staff physician of the center, the module team included at first a master's level nurse and two health assistants. During the later stages of the project, the nurse was replaced by a social worker who had had extensive experience in rehabilitation. The two health assistants were college graduates, one having majored in psychology and the other in sociology.

Module D was established in an urban community where home services were offered by a county agency and two private agencies. The module was attached to an ambulatory clinic that was administered by the same agency that administered Module C. The module professionals were a registered nurse and a family physician in private practice who had formerly been associated with the clinic. Both of the health assistants had had training in licensed practical nurse programs, and both spoke Spanish.

Module E was located in a rural community that had one home care program based in the county health department. This module was located initially in the health center of a public housing unit for elderly persons. Subsequently, the module was transferred to the county's medical care facility and was administered by the director of social services department. Module team members included a physician who was chief of staff at a local hospital, a nurse with rehabilitation expertise, and two health assistants. One health assistant was a licensed practical nurse, and the other had previously received some practical nurse training. (Health assistants in all modules also participated in the training program for chronic disease home care that will be described in the next chapter.)

COMPARISON OF URBAN AND RURAL PEOPLE

People selected for the study from urban and rural locations differed significantly by statistical test. As reported in Chapter 6, this difference did not bias the analyses of effects in the study, since our process of randomization assigned similar proportions of both urban and rural persons to each study group. Percentage figures in the following description are based on 449 people in urban locations and 425 in rural locations. The classifications and measures used were defined in Chapter 3.

The rural population included a larger proportion of older people than did the urban group—i.e., people seventy-five years or older. About one of every four urban persons (23%) and one of every three rural persons (37%) were seventy-five years or older. Black participants represented 18% of the urban group and only 4% of the rural group. Relatedly, the urban group included more people who were in the most dependent category of economic functioning (17%) as measured by the Index of Economic Dependence and in the lowest social class (23%) as measured by the Hollingshead Index. The respective proportions for rural people were 12% maximally dependent in economic functioning and 14% in the lowest social class. Although the proportions of widows and widowers did not differ remarkably between urban and rural people, more in the urban group were single (17% divorced, separated, or never married among urban people and 11% among rural people). A low degree of social involvement was more common in the urban group.

The health status of urban and rural people differed both in terms of the kinds of diseases and the amount of dependence in basic self-care activities. Whereas one-twelfth of rural persons (8%) had neoplasms, the percentage among urban persons was one-seventh (14%). Rural people, on the other hand, had more circulatory disease or diabetes (50% among the rural and 38% among the urban). Multiple dependencies in basic activities of daily living were twice as frequent in the urban group. Thus, 51% of those in the urban group had 3-6 areas of dependence as measured by the Index of Independence in Activities of Daily Living, while the corresponding percentage among rural people was 25%. Relatedly, those in the urban group had more days of bed disability, as demonstrated by the fact that about two-thirds in the urban group were disabled in bed for 7–14 days in a given two-week period, while less than one-half in the rural group had this amount of bed disability. By statistical test, significant differences between urban and rural groups were not observed with regard to sex, household composition, social desolation, and residence of person who gave personal assistance.

Chapter 5

MODULE SERVICE

Anne Cunningham
Joseph Papsidero
Ruth Clausen
Mary Wierenga

Module service was delivered by a mobile and flexible team oriented to services in the home. The physician, nurse or social worker, and health assistant used an interdisciplinary approach to identify patient problems, prepare a care plan, and define service activities, all of which were carefully and systematically documented and monitored.

The specific service performed by the team were evaluation-and care-centered. Evaluation-centered functions provided a profile that included a refined definition of disease, functional level, associated health problems, and appropriate objectives. Care-centered functions were service actions enabling achievement of objectives related to prevention, treatment, health maintenance, and rehabilitation. These service actions included assessment, management, referral, follow-up, and follow-through, as defined below.

1. Assessment is a systematic and continuing interdisciplinary process in which team members evaluate the total person, family, and environment, through observation and measurement of change in physical, psychological, economic, and social characteristics. These data are used to formulate a problem list and a continuing care plan for each problem.

2. Management is the active implementation of the continuing care plan, with specific consideration given to rehabilitation or restorative services, health maintenance, primary care, health education, prevention of complications or illnesses, and other approaches that improve or maintain function, stabilize medical status, and keep the patient at home.

3. Referral is the utilization and coordination of health care resources in the community to meet the needs of the person and family and facilitate management goals.

4. Follow-up and follow-through are actions which insure that the referral process was successfully completed and the needs of the patient were met.

SERVICE ROLES

The roles of each member of the team in performing the functions described above are identified in the following outline.

A. Physician

    1. Assessment

        a. Evaluated adequacy of medical information.

        b. Relayed orders for medications and treatment regimen from attending physician.

        c. Assessed with social worker or nurse the behavioral skills required for medical management.

        d. Assessed the type of instruction necessary for family members or others responsible for care.

        e. Discussed general condition of the ill person and assisted in developing a problem list.

    2. Management

        a. Provided information on disease condition, underlying physiology, effect of care on prognosis, and secondary prevention.

      b.   Gave medical approval of team proposal for care and management.

  3. Referral

Evaluated any specialized health care needs in management of the disease and referred to appropriate medical channels.

  4. Follow-up/Follow-through

Provided continuing channel of communication to specialized medical referral to assess adequacy of referral care.

B. Nurse or Social Worker

  1. Assessment
      a.   Performed initial assessment of ill person.
      b.   Assisted in team assessment and understanding of significant social, emotional, and economic factors related to person's care.
      c.   Assisted in organizing person's module service record for continuing assessment of the case management.

  2. Management
      a.   Initiated introduction of the module to the person and family.
      b.   Assumed primary responsibility in developing problem list and management plan.
      c.   Provided expertise in rehabilitation nursing techniques and in interpretation of home care nursing orders.
      d.   Offered ongoing supervision of health assistant's activities.

  3. Referral

Relayed knowledge regarding community resources (health, financial, recreational, education) available to person and family; referred to appropriate agency.

  4. Follow-up/Follow-through

Assured that referral process was adequately completed; provided feedback on success of that process.

C. Health Assistant

  1. Assessment

    a. Provided ongoing assessment of person during periodic home care visits; also assessed family situation, social and economic setting, and any other factors affecting person's progress and care.
    b. Provided assessment of any family members that needed professional care.

  2. Management

    a. Relayed information about home visits to the team in the Problem Oriented Medical Record format for use in matching person's needs and resources in home environment to the other team member's skills.
    b. Helped in preparation of health assistant problem-oriented task list.
    c. Performed the bulk of direct service to person and family in the home.
    d. Educated person and family for self-management.
    e. Provided some transportation for person.

  3. Referral

    Assisted in referrals to other agencies (social, educational, health care agencies according to person's assessed need).

  4. Follow-up/Follow-through

    Through follow-up home visits, provided continued feedback on success of referral programs in meeting the specific needs of person.

Data collection and initial assessment of the person were conducted by the module's nurse or social worker upon the patient's entry into module care. Social, cultural, economic, and demographic information, prior and current health status and medical care, family, and home conditions, both physical and social, were assessed. This information was obtained with the primary care physician and referral physicians, interviews with the person and family or close friends, and observation of the home conditions. The assessment was recorded on forms and updated throughout the provision of care. Care was instituted as promptly as possible to insure continuity of health services. The module physician established initial contact with the person's primary care physician to explain module care, learn about recommended home care regimens, identify the specific nature of the relationship between module and primary care physician, and establish an ongoing method of communication.

All team members participated in the initial identification of personal and family problems and in planning of home care activities. The module physician clarified biomedical aspects of disease and informed the other team members regarding the implications of the physical assessments of the patient and probable course of illness. Team members used the physician's input to assist in problem-solving and care management activities. The module nurse or social worker developed the written plan for care and determined the level of intensity of service, including the specific tasks to be carried out by health assistants. Significantly, the module nurse or social worker introduced the health assistant to the patient and family as a professional extender at the point when the care management process was initiated.

Following the initial gathering of data, team members discussed the information at regularly scheduled team conferences. In the case conferences, as in the ongoing management process, each member of the module team had a clear role. The management process relied mainly upon the health assistant's continued assessment during each home visit. The health assistant observed the person in activities of daily living and in social interactions, and talked with the person, family, and other care givers regarding progress. The health assistant recorded this information and reported it to module team members at the regular team conferences, unless immediate action was required. Sometimes the team requested that the health assistant make specific observations on subsequent visits and report these at the next team conference. For example, the health assistant may have been asked to test the patient for mental status using a standard measure of mental functioning, conduct a range-of-motion test, test for muscle strength, measure some aspect of social interaction, or observe other members of the family and their health care needs.

HEALTH ASSISTANT PERFORMANCE AND TRAINING

1. Services Performed by the Health Assistant

   The activities of the health assistant represented the extension of selected skills of the physician, nurse, social worker, and rehabilitation therapists, such as occupational therapists, physical therapists, speech therapists, and audiologists. The objectives of health assistant activities pertaining to rehabilitation were to assist the patient to achieve and maintain an optimal level of physical functioning and to prevent, as far as possible, secondary complications of the disease process. In general, the rehabilitation functions focused on activities of daily living: bathing, dressing, going to the toilet, walking, feeding, etc. The health assistant provided or taught others to provide therapeutic exercises to increase muscular strength and coordination so that the person was better able to carry out activities of daily living and prevent or delay physical deterioration. The health assistant also performed household management tasks intended to provide a safe and healthful home environment and increase the person's mobility—as, for example, physical modification of the home to accommodate loss in physical functioning, and light housekeeping as necessary until other more permanent arrangements could be made.

   Other health assistant activities were designed to promote social functioning and were also varied and individualized. A therapeutic relationship was established with the person and family that enabled improved communication of concerns, social problems, and conflicts that may have interfered with the person's care and rehabilitation. Discussion about the disease process was facilitated to increase the patient's understanding of and adaptation to disease, disability, and the care process. Support in the terminal stages of the disease was provided when necessary. In addition, the health assistant aided the patient in developing greater social awareness by direct interaction, helped the patient and family participate in community activities and find productive, enjoyable ways to use leisure time. The health assistant sought to alleviate economic problems by suitable referrals and made arrangements for housing if the patient's living situation was unsafe or inadequate for the person's or family's needs.

2.   Training for Service

The goal of the instructional program for health assistants was to provide a systematic learning experience by which specialized knowledge, attitudes, and skills were acquired. Thus, the health assistants were prepared to (a) provide assistance in selected patient care management functions in the home, (b) perform on-going assessment of patient functioning, and (c) help the chronically ill individual and his/her family to cope realistically with health-related and social problems.

The instructional program for health assistants was implemented in two phases over a nine-month, three-quarter period. Phase I, the "pre-service" phase, required health assistants to enroll in selected introductory community college courses. These courses provided instruction in basic medical terminology, anatomy, physiology, nursing, and other topics considered to be consistent with overall objectives. Phase II, the "in-service" phase, provided a specialized field experience offered by the faculty of a Cadre Training Unit, a group organized as a training and continuing care module. This phase required the health assistant to increase knowledge and skills about care of the chronically ill and to demonstrate these in the home under supervision. Phase I and Phase II overlapped midway during the nine-month period. Upon successful completion of the course of study, health assistants were granted a certificate.

As a parallel activity, the professional development seminars for health care professionals were also implemented during the nine-month period, and required increasing time commitment up to eight hours a week. The physicians, nurses, and social workers selected for each module attended seminars related to professional problem-solving, team functioning, and the pattern and policies of module service.

A third phase of the educational program began when the health assistants and module professionals started a three-month period of service in the host agency, as a team. Team performance as well as individual performance were assessed. A program of continuing orientation in which the educational processes described above were reinforced and evaluated was then initiated and continued through the study period.

ILLUSTRATIONS OF CARE IN THE HOME

The observational and helping activities of health assistants in the home were centered upon such areas as patient behavior in following prescribed treatment, emotional response to treatment, improvement or lack of improvement in health status, level of independence of functioning in activities of daily living, early detection of new problems or complications associated with existing problems, and socioeconomic problems. Various aspects of these activities and functions are presented in the case illustrations that follow.

1. Assessment and Care Management

Mrs. H., a 46-year-old woman, had been diagnosed with multiple sclerosis six years before being referred to module service. When she was initially assessed by the module, she had been highly dependent in the activities of daily living (ADL) for about three years. The dependencies included: (a) bathing —washed face occasionally, daughter bathed; (b) dressing— daughter helped with nightgown, only got dressed when going out, which was infrequent; (c) toilet—used bedpan which daughter emptied; (d) transfer—required two people to lift her into chair, three people to help her into the car; (e) feeding—fed self lying flat in bed, stated she was too weak to sit up; and (f) walking—used wheelchair but often spent most of the day in bed. All of her joints had some instability and there were muscle weakness, wasting, and atrophy. She experienced spasms in the lower extremities, and weakness in the upper extremities. The upper extremities were graded as poor. She also had vision, sensation, bladder, and bowel impairment. The module team arranged to have Mrs. H. admitted to a rehabilitation center for evaluation and therapy. They helped arrange for the daughter to visit and to be taught the elements of the care plan by the rehabilitation therapist. The nurse in the rehabilitation center and the nurse in Mrs. H.'s module communicated frequently to provide continuity of care.

When Mrs. H. returned to her home, the health assistant continued the treatment prescribed by the rehabilitation center. She continued teaching the daughter management techniques regarding exercises and diet, and continued to supervise these and Mrs. H.'s activity of daily living on every visit. Four months after the health assistant's initial visit, Mrs. H.'s level of independence in the ADL was: (a) bathing—bathed self sitting on the side of bed, daughter did perineal area; (b) dressing—dressed self, daughter got clothes out; (c) toileting—used bedpan, stayed in bed in the morning when taking diuretic; (d) transfer—transferred self to wheelchair and returned to bed, one person assisted into the car; (e) continence—incontinence was rare; (f) feeding—fed self at kitchen table; and (g) mobility—able to do simple wheelchair maneuvering.

With this increase in functional ability, Mrs. H. began increasing her social contacts. She was able to go shopping, fishing, and attend church. Her anxiety decreased. In only four months of module service, the team assessed Mrs. H.'s health as improved substantially both mentally and physically.

Mrs. H. maintained the above level of independence in ADL for the next two and a half years. The health assistant continued to provide support, encouragement, and supervision through this time. When the health assistant found that Mrs. H.'s legs were becoming stronger, the team decided to ask for physical therapy re-evaluation consultation. Mrs. H. started to stand with a walker for five minutes. The health assistant also maintained Mrs. H. through the death of her daughter and assisted her in obtaining housekeeping services with help from the Department of Social Services.

2.   Referral

Mrs. B., a 68-year-old woman, had severe rheumatoid arthritis and had undergone seven operations, including left hip surgery, in the two and a half years before module service. Her husband also had several chronic diseases. The B.'s owned their own small home, which had a front ramp to accommodate her wheelchair. However, several structural problems were evident, such as a kitchen counter top which was too high and a small kitchen area that prevented Mrs. B. from turning her wheelchair around. Mrs. B. needed help with home management, but Mr. B. did not at that time know how to help. After Mrs. B. was discharged from the hospital the Visiting Nurse Association provided Mrs. B. with skilled nursing care for approximately one month. The health assistant and the visiting nurse scheduled their visits on alternate days so that Mrs. B. had help walking and exercising each day. The Visiting Nurse Association also provided a home health aide for one month for meal preparation and light housekeeping. After this period, the health assistant made arrangements with the County Department of Social Service for a part-time housekeeper. During this time the health assistant helped Mr. B. to assume some of the household tasks, to learn how to schedule housework, and to cook breakfast. Mrs. B. was taught how to transfer herself and to use a commode placed next to her bed.

The health assistant helped the B.'s to decrease their social isolation. An adopt-a-grandparent program provided a young volunteer approximately once a week. Mrs. B. began to write letters for a local association of retired people. The health assistant continued to work with Mrs. B. on walking and exercises, helping her to progress to platform crutches. The increased mobility, although still quite limited, allowed Mrs. B. to be more independent, and when spring arrived she was able to go outdoors more frequently.

3. Follow-up and Follow-through

Mrs. D., a 74-year-old Cherokee Indian, had widespread rectal cancer. She lived with her son and daughter-in-law. The health assistant talked to the family about Mrs. D.'s future care and their fears about coping with the situation. They talked about the possibility of placing Mrs. D. in a nursing home when the care became too difficult for the family to handle. The health assistant assured the family that she would do what she could to assist in Mrs. D.'s care and would visit more often when her condition required more care. As Mrs. D.'s condition deteriorated, the health assistant increased the frequency of her visits from once a week to twice a week. Mrs. D. called the health assistant at 8:00 p.m. one evening, complaining of vaginal bleeding. She was alone and frightened. The health assistant called an ambulance and then went to Mrs. D.'s home. Mrs. D.'s grandaughter arrived shortly afterwards and together they tried to calm Mrs. D. The health assistant notified Mrs. D.'s physician that she would be arriving at the hospital. The health assistant made follow-up visits to see Mrs. D. in the hospital.

Six months later, Mrs. D. was admitted to an extended care facility. The health assistant had helped the family make arrangements, but left the actual decision up to them. The assistant's note in the chart at the time of Mrs. D.'s admission to the facility read "she was very alert and seemed to be content in her new surroundings."

MODULE CASE LOAD AND COST OF SERVICE

Patient data were recorded, using the problem-oriented medical record format. Initial lists of problems, medications, and care plans were complete. Other forms related to patient care planning were updated through continuing assessment of the person's problems and needs. A special form was used to record each health assistant visit to the home, either alone or accompanied by the nurse or social worker. The data from these forms provided a description of the case load and the amount of time spent on different service activities in the home. The total module case load included persons in the study as well as other family members in the same residence who were not in the study. In order to more completely describe the team service, the remaining discussion will refer to the total module case load as the persons in the study as well as any family members receiving service.

Total visit time was reported as the sum of visit time in the home, traveling time, and charting time. This averaged approximately eighty minutes for each visit (Table 5.1). When the monthly averages of visit-related time for home visits for each site were compared over the sampled period of fourteen months, there were no appreciable differences over time.

The time spent in different service activities in the home is shown in Table 5.2. This data was obtained from the Health Assistant Activity Sheet. A high proportion of service time in the home was spent in problem assessment and direct assistance. Examination of the service records indicated that in the sample period, 91% of the

Figure 5.1

Module Case Load and Time Spent in Home Visits*

Variable	Urban Modules		Rural Modules		
	A	D	B	C	E
Average case load	27	22 (30**)	36	32	20 (23**)
Average number of visits per month	67	98	106	78	79
Average number of visits per case per month	2.5	4.4	2.9	2.4	4.0
Average time spent in home visit (min.)	44	53	44	40	48
Average charting time (min.)	15	13	11	9	10
Average time spent on travel to and from home (min.)	18	26	18	25	19
Average total visit-related time (min.)	77	92	73	74	77

* November 1974 to December 1975
** Average at full operation.

visits included at least some attention to medical supervision, 70% involved some assistance with interpersonal relations, 48% concerned adjustment to illness, and 39% included home management and nutrition.

In assessing the resources used in providing module service, a critical issue was the determination of the number of patients a module with a given level of resources could serve effectively. Obviously, the more patients served, the lower the cost per patient. It was felt that the actual number of patients served by the modules in the project did not reflect the number of patients that could be served by a module operating at full capacity. There were several

Table 5.2

Comparison Among Modules of the Per Cent of Home
Visit Time in Various Activities*

Service Activity in the Home	Urban Modules		Rural Modules		
	A %	D %	B %	C %	E %
Problem Assessment	37.1	22.7	47.2	56.2	42.4
Education of Patient	23.9	2.3	2.9	2.2	4.6
Education of Family	3.7	2.3	2.1	5.0	3.4
Direct Assistance	19.5	44.2	41.8	12.3	28.1
Transportation of Patient	3.2	7.3	3.1	9.7	7.2
Referral	2.4	0.1	0.4	2.8	1.4
Consultations	3.1	0.5	0.4	3.0	1.8
Other Case-Related Activity	6.4	20.3	1.8	7.0	11.1
Other Activity	0.6	0.1	0.1	1.6	0.1
Total Percent**	99.9	99.8	99.8	99.8	100.1

* November, 1974 to December, 1975
** Deviation from 100% due to rounding error.

reasons for this. The health assistant was a new type of manpower performing new types of services in the home and there was no past experience to help in judging how large a case load a health assistant could handle while maintaining adequate quality of care. It was decided that the modules should try to limit the case load to forty patients, twenty per health assistant. The experience with this project has shown that the twenty patients per health assistant limit could be increased.

Since it was felt that the actual case loads were reduced because of the above mentioned factors, it would be misleading to use only those figures to determine per patient costs. Two other figures, besides the actual case loads, were used. These are estimates of case load capacity as made by the module administrator and by the module nurse or social worker assuming the same average of 2.9 visits to each patient every month.

The lowest figure was the actual reported case load, an average of thirty cases per module. The administrator's average estimate of case load capacity was forty-one cases while the nurse or social worker's estimate of capacity was fifty cases per module.

It was found that the pattern of module costs was similar in all five modules. Overall personnel costs represented 77% of total module operating costs. This figure included the salaries for a quarter-time physician, a part-time administrator, a half-time nurse or social worker, and two full-time health assistants. The health assistant salaries and fringe benefits alone represented 36% of the total module operating costs. Nonpersonnel operating costs covered the majority of the remaining expenses, approximately 23% of the total.

The costs of resources used per person per month for module service was determined by dividing the costs of module operations by the estimates of case load capacity. Using the actual reported case load, the average monthly cost per person for all modules was $113. Using the administrators' estimate of module capacity, the average cost would have been $82 per person per month. The estimates of the module nurse or social worker who was most intimately involved in providing the service indicated that this figure might be reduced to $68.

The cost per visit figures also used the three case load estimates. The nurse or social worker estimate of capacity case load was the lowest estimate of cost per visit at $24 per visit. The hourly operating cost per visit ranged from $8.59 to $11.79, with an average of $10.09.

CONSULTATION TO COMMUNITIES ON CERTIFICATION AND REIMBURSEMENT OF MODULE SERVICE

A long-term objective of this project was to assist host agencies in exploring ways of obtaining certification of and reimbursement for module service. In this process, our community organization specialist, along with other project staff, prepared detailed analyses of current regulations, documentation of alternative ways of financing home care, and other materials that the host agency could use in seeking certification or in recommending changes in regulations concerning the eligibility of module services for third party payments.

The issue of reimbursement for module services was crucial. Regulations for home health care providers favored skilled nursing care reimbursement. Personal and social care delivered in the home setting, a characteristic of module care, needed to be legitimized in the eyes of third party payors. It could not realistically become an integral part of the host facility's program otherwise.

The module administrators were encouraged to seek certification as providers of basic care rather than providers of only "skilled nursing" as required in present federal regulations for Medicare and Medicaid. At the time of termination of federal funds for module service, one agency integrated the module team into its own service system. This agency had the advantage of already being a certified home health care provider and offering the "skilled nursing" that the conditions of participation presently require.

REFERENCE

Weed, L. L. 1970. *Medical Records, Medical Education, and Patient Care: The Problem-Oriented Record as a Basic Tool.* Cleveland: The Press of Case Western Reserve University.

Chapter 6

THE STUDY GROUPS

Sidney Katz
Sister Mary Honora Kroger

Comparability of study groups is an important issue in any randomized study. Therefore, it is necessary to describe study groups in terms of characteristics and factors considered important on the basis of theory and previous experience. In addition to their use in evaluating the randomization process, such characteristics served as a basis for constructing classifications which were used in analyses of service effects and in discussion of policy implications.

In the "real-life" implementation of this type of social experiment, services may be assigned at random but cannot be forced upon or applied to all who are so assigned. Total or partial nonacceptance may occur for reasons such as the rights of individuals, provider resistance within the community, and absence of common viewpoints about the need for services. As a result, variations occur in acceptance and intensity of service, posing problems with regard to the final judgments that are made about the service program's effectiveness. Since acceptance and intensity of module service must be considered when results are interpreted, we also describe these characteristics in this chapter.

CHARACTERISTICS OF PARTICIPANTS IN
THE STUDY GROUPS

Table 6.1, 6.2, and 6.3, present detailed information about those who were referred to module service and those who were not referred to such service.

Participants ranged in age from forty-five to ninety-eight years

Table 6.1

Identifying Characteristics

	Referred to Module Service	Not Referred to Module Service
	(numbers of persons)	
Age		
45–64 years	171	173
65–74 years	137	132
75 years and older	130	131
Sex		
Men	177	175
Women	261	261
Marital Status		
Married	223	218
Widow or widower	120	143
Divorced or separated	41	28
Never married	26	24
Unknown	28	23
Location		
Urban	226	223
Rural	212	213
House Composition		
Lived alone	88	83
Lived with others	322	325
Unknown	28	28
Residence of Person Who Gives Personal Assistance		
Lived with participant	231	250
Lived apart from participant	173	157
No person	6	4
Unknown	28	25

as they entered the study, as shown in Table 6.1. About three of every ten were seventy-five years old or older, and a similar number were sixty-five to seventy-four years old. As might be expected in a relatively aged group, the larger number were women (60%). Slightly more than half of the participants were married, and one-third were widows or widowers. Those who were referred to module service did not differ significantly relative to age, sex, and marital status from those who were not referred to module service (probability greater than 0.05 by chi-square test).

Participants were about equally distributed between communities

Table 6.2

Social and Economic Characteristics

	Referred to Module Service	Not Referred to Module Service
	(numbers of persons)	
Social Class (Hollingshead Scale)*		
Classes I, II, III, and IV	249	244
Class V	139	153
Unknown	50	39
Index of Economic Dependence*		
Independent (Class 1)	38	31
Partly dependent (Classes 2 & 3)	300	284
Dependent (Class 4)	49	60
Unknown	51	61
Payment for Health Care		
Private funds	216	210
Public assistance	101	110
Unknown	121	116
Social Role and Activities*		
Much involvement	122	127
Moderate involvement	280	274
Uninvolved	7	10
Unknown	29	25
Social Desolation*		
No personal loss events	222	220
1–4 personal loss events	122	131
Unknown	94	85

* See Chapter 3 for definitions of classes and for references.

classified as urban (population of 220,000 to 420,000) and rural (population of 20,000 to 45,000). Only one of five lived alone. Among those who received nonprofessional personal care, three of every five received such care principally from someone who lived in the same residence. With regard to location, household composition, and residence of the principal nonprofessional person who gave care, those who were referred to module service did not differ significantly from those who were not referred to module service (probability greater than 0.05 by chi-square test).

Considering social position as derived by the Hollingshead Index, about one-third of the study participants were in Class V, defined as unskilled or semiskilled workers (Table 6.2). Executives and professionals of all types comprised only 5% of the total sample, a figure that was considerably smaller than the 12.4% found in a sample of households in New Haven (Hollingshead and Redlich 1958). The observation that many participants in the present study had limited economic resources was also supported by their distribution according to the Index of Economic Dependence and by the number who received public assistance to pay for health care. The Index of Economic Dependence is based on employment status, home ownership, and source of economic support. Among the participants, 91% either were unemployed, did not receive assistance from public agencies, or did not own their own homes. One-third received public assistance to pay for health care. Most of the participants were not completely independent in these terms, and one of every seven was completely dependent.

Social role and activities reflect the degree of interaction with the social environment and, thus, the available resources that can be of assistance in case of need. As a measure of such interaction, about one-third of the participants were involved in many activities with spouse, family members, friends, and work (Table 6.2). Almost two-thirds were moderately involved, and only 2% were uninvolved. More than one-third of the participants had experienced recent losses, a group to whom we applied the term social desolate or deprived. Such losses included one or more of the following: discontinuance of work or homemaking, and significant persons who moved away or died. With regard to the aspects of economic and social functioning that we reviewed, those who were referred to module service did not differ significantly from those who were not referred to module service (probability greater than 0.05 by chi-square test).

As an expected result of the eligibility criteria for this study, all participants selected had chronic diseases. About three-fourths had

Table 6.3

Health and Mental Status

	Referred to Module Service	Not Referred to Module Service
	(numbers of persons)	
Principal Diseases*		
Circulatory system	153	153
Neoplasms	51	47
Musculoskeletal system and connective tissue	46	35
Endocrine, metabolic, and nutritional	35	40
Respiratory	37	34
Digestive	24	31
Other	87	86
Unknown	5	10
Activities of Daily Living (Index of ADL)*		
Independent in all 6 activities	130	140
Dependent in 1 or 2 activities	105	127
Dependent in 3 to 6 activities	172	143
Unknown	31	26
Severity of Illness**		
0 to 2 ADL dependencies and low risk disease	93	102
0 to 2 ADL dependencies and high risk disease	138	156
3 to 6 ADL dependencies and any disease	171	142
Unknown	36	36
Orientation (Kahn's MSQ)*		
8 to 10 correct answers	367	367
0 to 7 correct answers	40	43
Unknown	31	26

* See Chapter 3 for definitions of classes and for references.
** See text of this chapter (Chapter 6) for definitions and for references.

diseases of the circulatory system, neoplasms, diabetes, or diseases of the musculoskeletal system and connective tissue (Table 6.3). Of these conditions, diseases of the circulatory system were the most common, affecting one-third of the participants. This finding is consistent with the observation that heart conditions are the leading causes of activity limitation among persons in the United States who are similar in age to the study participants (DHEW 1973). With regard to disability, two-thirds of those in the present study had some loss of capacity to perform one or more of six major activities of daily living (bathing, dressing, going to toilet, transferring, continence, feeding). Two of every five participants were limited in at least three of the six functions. As a measure of severity of illness, we established a "profile" for each individual, consisting of a rating for that individual's disability status and a rating for her/his disease status (Commission on Chronic Illness 1957; Akpom et al. 1974). Three severity grades were thus defined. The least severely ill group included persons who were dependent in zero to two of the six activities of daily living and had diseases that were considered to be of relatively low risk. The next severity grade included those who were dependent in zero to two activities of daily living and had diseases that were considered to be relatively high risk. The most severe grade included persons who were dependent in three or more of the six activities of daily living, regardless of diagnosis. Relatively "high risk" diseases included degenerative diseases of the cardio-vascular-renal, central nervous, and pulmonary systems, as well as neoplasms and diabetes. Other diseases were included in the "low risk" class. When classified according to these three grades of severity, 24% were in the least severely ill group; 37% were moderately severely ill; and 39% were in the most severely ill group. As an indicator of mental function, Kahn's Mental Status Questionnaire revealed that 90% of the participants correctly answered eight to ten questions about orientation with regard to time, place, and person (Table 6.3). Participants who were referred to module service did not differ significantly as to disease, disability, severity of illness, and mental orientation, from those who were not referred to module service (probability greater than 0.05 by chi-square test).

As described above, identifying physical, psychological and social characteristics did not differ significantly between study groups, thus, demonstrating the effectiveness of randomization.

INTENSITY OF SERVICE

Although services were assigned in a random manner, patients could not be forced to accept such services; thus, services were not always accepted and, when accepted, were accepted with varying degrees of intensity. We established three grades of intensity, related to the measures used in our previous home care experiment (Katz et al. 1972). Persons in the first or lowest level of intensity received health assistant visits for a total period of two months or less during the first six months of the study. Included also in the first or low level were those who did not accept service at all. Included in the second or medium level of intensity were individuals who were visited by health assistants during at least three of the first six months and who received less than one visit per ten days on the average. The third or highest level of intensity included those who were visited during at least three of the first six months and who received one or more visits per ten days in the average.

The proportions of patients in the low, medium, and high intensity groups were 66%, 19%, and 15%, respectively (Table 6.4). The validity of these classes is represented in Tables 6.4 and 6.5. All participants in the low intensity class were visited during two or fewer of the first six months, while all in the medium and high intensity classes were visited during more than two months. Of those in the medium intensity class, one-third were visited during three to four months, and two-thirds were visited during five to six months. Correspondingly, of those in the high intensity group, 95% were visited during five to six months. The number of consecutive months of visits paralleled the total number of months of visits for each of the three groups, respectively. Two-thirds of those in the high intensity group averaged at least one visit per week during four to six months (four or more visits per month), while none in the two lower intensity groups experienced this frequency of visiting.

We examined changes in the intensity of service between the

first and second six months of the study among those who lived beyond the first six months (Table 6.5). We found that the intensity of visits was the same during the second six months as during the first six months for 87% of the participants. The intensity of visits decreased during the second six months in 11%, while intensity increased in 2%. The aforementioned evaluations demonstrate the validity of the intensity classes in terms of the duration of visits, frequency of visits, and consistency of the classes between the first and second six months of the study.

The reasons for nonacceptance of service by those who were referred to module service are presented in Table 6.6. These reasons were considered in terms of perceived need, acknowledging that perception varies with respect to the following factors: utility of the services offered, needs of the individual, supports available to the

Table 6.4

Intensity of Service

	Intensity Class*		
	Low	Medium	High
Numbers of Persons (n)	284	83	64
Months Visited During First 6 months (per cent of n)			
0 to 2 months	100.0	0.0	0.0
3 to 4 months	0.0	33.7	4.7
5 to 6 months	0.0	66.2	95.3
Consecutive Months Visited (per cent of n)			
0 to 2 months	100.0	0.0	0.0
3 to 4 months	0.0	33.7	4.7
5 to 6 months	0.0	66.2	95.3
Months of 4 or More Visits Per Month (per cent of n)			
0 to 1 month	100.0	84.3	0.0
2 to 3 months	0.0	15.6	37.5
4 to 6 months	0.0	0.0	62.6

* See text of this chapter (Chapter 6) for definitions of intensity classes. For 7 of the 438 participants who were referred to module service, the intensity class could not be measured.

Table 6.5

Changes in Intensity of Service Between First and
Second Six Months of Study

		*Intensity of Service During First Six Months**				
		*Low***	*Medium*	*High*	*Unknown*	*Totals*
		(numbers of persons)				
Intensity of Service During Second Six Months*	Low	271	17	7	—	295
	Medium	1	47	20	—	68
	High	—	8	29	—	37
	Deceased	12	7	6	—	25
	Unknown	—	4	2	7	13
	Totals	284	83	64	7	438

* See text of this chapter (Chapter 6) for definitions of intensity classes.
** Using this column as an example, the table is read as follows: of the total 284 persons who received low intensity of service during the first six months, 271 remained at that level of intensity, 1 received medium intensity and 12 died.

patient, and the type of person making the judgment. Based on these considerations, the reasons for nonacceptance fell into five general categories. Four per cent of the refusals were based on the view that institutional care was needed. For another 11%, organized home services other than module service were selected. For 24% the reason for nonacceptance was the stated view that family or friends could adequately serve the needs of the patients. The family member or friend available to give service was a person with health care provider training in more than 20% of the latter group of sixty patients. Reasons other than the above accounted for 45% of the refusals and were expressed most often by the patient or by the patient's personal physician. For 16% of the instances of non-acceptance, the perceived need could not be determined because contact could not be established, because a reason was not given, or because the recorded information about need was unclear.

As indicated earlier, intensity of service was used as a measure of the degree of acceptance or lack of acceptance of module service. In order to further evaluate reasons for acceptance and nonac-

Table 6.6

Reasons Expressed for Nonacceptance of Module Service

Reason	Number of Persons
Institutional care needed	10
Home service agency other than module service selected	27
Need covered by family or friends	60
Without provider training (47 participants)	
With provider training (13 participants)	
No need for module service	111
Decision made by physician (27 participants)	
Decision made by participant (80 participants)	
Decision made by spouse, other family member, or friend (4 participants)	
Perception of need not known	41
Total	249

ceptance, the attributes of people who clearly accepted service (medium and high intensity groups) were compared with the attributes of those who did not accept service. This comparison also helped us search for self-selection factors that should be taken into account in order to avoid biased interpretations of the results of the study. We compared the two groups in terms of the characteristics and classifications that were used in the analyses of effects. The characteristics are the same identifying and physical, psychological, and social factors that are displayed in Tables 6.1, 6.2, and 6.3. Similarly, we compared the persons who did not accept service with those who were not referred to module service (the control group).

When compared with persons who did not accept service, participants in the medium and high intensity service groups included more women, more who were economically dependent, and more who were receiving public assistance (probability less than 0.05 by chi-square test). Relatedly, when compared to persons who did not accept service, patients who were not referred to module service (the control group) included more who were economically dependent and more who were receiving public assistance (probability less than 0.05 by chi-square test). Thus, the acceptance or demand for services was influenced by economic status and sex.

REFERENCES

Akpom, C. A., Katz, S., and Densen, P. M. 1973. Methods of classifying disability and severity of illness in ambulatory care patients. *Medical Care* (Supplement) 11:125–131.

Commission on Chronic Illness. 1957. *Chronic Illness in the United States. Vol. IV, Chronic Illness in a Large City.* Cambridge: Harvard University Press.

Hollingshead, A. B., and Redlich, F. C. 1958. *Social Class and Mental Illness.* New York: John Wiley & Sons, Inc.

Katz, S., Ford, A. B., Downs, T. D., Adams, M., and Rusby, D. I. 1972. *Effects of Continued Care: A Study of Chronic Illness in the Home.* DHEW Publication No. (HSM) 73–3010. U.S. Government Printing Office, Washintgon, D.C.

U.S. Department of Health, Education, and Welfare. 1973. Limitation of activity due to chronic conditions, United States, 1969 and 1970. *Vital and Health Statistics Data from the National Health Survey.* DHEW Publication No. (HSM) 73–1506, Series 10, No. 80, U.S. Government Printing Office, Washington, D.C.

Chapter 7

EFFECTS OF
MODULE SERVICE

Joseph Papsidero
Michael Branson
C. Amechi Akpom

As reported, persons who were referred to module service did not differ significantly from persons in the control group who were not referred to module service. This statement is based on comparisons of physical, psychological, and socio-demographic characteristics which previous studies had shown to be important prognostic factors for similar people. Since the two study groups were expected to be heterogeneous in terms of these characteristics, we anticipated that such variability might obscure the effects of module service. Therefore, for the purpose of refined analysis, we defined eighteen homogeneous subgroups. For each of the eighteen groups we separately analyzed effects among (1) those who clearly used module services which we defined as medium and high intensity of service, and (2) those who accepted minimal module services or none at all, defined as low intensity of service.

Figure 7.1 summarizes the specific classifications that were used

Figure 7.1

Classifications Used in Analyses of Effects

Study Groups	Homogeneous Subgroups	Outcomes
Referred to Module Service	Age	Activities of Daily Living
low intensity	45–64 years	Walking
medium intensity	65–74 years	Mobility
high intensity	75 years and older	Disability Days
Not Referred to Module Service	Social Class (Hollingshead)	Mortality
	classes I–IV	Contentment
	class V	Social Role and Activities
	Social Role and Activities	Orientation
	much involvement	Observation and Clear Thinking
	moderate involvement	Economic Dependence
	uninvolved	Institutionalization
	Social Desolation	
	no personal loss events	
	1–4 personal loss events	
	Primary Diagnosis	
	low risk	
	high risk	
	Activities of Daily Living	
	dependent in 0–2 activities	
	dependent in 3–6 activities	

Figure 7.1 (Cont.)

Classifications Used in Analyses of Effects

Study Groups	Homogeneous Subgroups	Outcomes
	Severity of Illness	
	0–2 ADL dependencies and low risk disease	
	0–2 ADL dependencies and high risk disease	
	3–6 ADL dependencies and any disease*	
	Orientation (MSQ)	
	8–10 correct answers	
	0–7 correct answers	

* This variable is the same as "dependent in 3–6 activities" included in the preceding ADL classification.

in the analyses of effects. The classifications were the same as those used in the comparisons in Chapter 6. Our approach to functional classification has evolved over the past seventeen years and has been validated through epidemiologic and experimental studies of chronically ill disabled people. The measures used to arrive at these classifications are described in Chapter 3 and are widely accepted on the basis of current knowledge about their reliability and validity.

Conceptual issues related to measurement and interpretation were discussed in an earlier publication in which we observed: "Certain kinds of interpretations about patient well being are, of course, more acceptable than others, due to limitations of available measures. For some functions, such as walking and activities of daily living, we have precisely defined reproducible measures, while for other functions, such as social interaction and social adjustment, definitions and reproducibility of measures are limited. Another limitation is that currently available measures do not cover all the areas of functions included in the concept of comprehensive well being." (Katz et al. 1972).

In view of such constraints on interpretation, we applied the term "benefit" only to effects on physical and mental function. We referred to effects on social function as "changes." Consistent with our main hypothesis, a beneficial effect was defined as improvement *or* maintenance in function, not improvement alone; thus the term "benefit" was limited to circumstances in which we demonstrated that physical or mental deterioration among those who clearly used high or medium intensity module service was less frequent than deterioration among the people who were not referred to module service. Our use of such phrases as "more often associated," "occurred more frequently," "more frequently maintained or improved," "fewer deteriorations," "beneficial service effect," "more services," and "fewer admissions" are all based on demonstrated significance by statistical test within the limitations discussed below.

The statistically significant findings reported in this chapter are based on the application of a chi square test for independence. For each test, the data were arranged in a 2 by 2 contingency table and the chi square test statistic with the continuity correction was computed. The following describes this procedure, using as an example the observed twelve-month effects in activities of daily living (ADL) for populations of *High and Medium Service Intensity* vs. *Control.* For each person in the total experimental and in the total control group, ADL was measured at the beginning and end of a twelve-month interval; and the difference was computed. Each person was classified as deteriorated or non-deteriorated based on this difference, resulting in the following 2 by 2 table:

| *Group* | *Outcome* | | *Row* |
	Non-Deteriorated	*Deteriorated*	*Total*
Experimental	65	14	79
Control	181	26	207
Total	246	40	286

A chi square test statistic was then computed to see if group and outcome are independent in a statistical sense. Using our example, this is equivalent to testing the hypothesis that the percent of subjects with deterioration in ADL is equal in the experimental and the control group. The foregoing example describes the basic form of all statistical tests for 456 comparisons of data the results of which are reported in this chapter.

It should be noted that several other statistical approaches were considered. The chi square test was selected in part because it would provide data comparable to the Continued Care Study (Katz et al. 1972). One major limitation of this approach should be mentioned. In the tables and discussion that follow, chi square tests were repeatedly run at the 95% level. If any one test is considered separately, the significance level holds. However, when the tests are considered together, the 95% level is not maintained. One approach to this problem is to use multivariate statistical methods such as log-linear models (Feinberg 1977). The use of these advanced approaches in post-hoc analysis is currently being explored. However, it is anticipated that such analysis will not reverse any findings reported in this chapter.

Another limitation of the study is that nonacceptance of service could lead to the potential bias of self-selection. Thus, any generalizations beyond the specific subjects in this study must be made with caution.

In the description of results that follows, we report statistically significant differences between the total service and control study groups. We also report statistically significant differences found among the eighteen subgroups as listed in Figure 7.1. In addition, we report findings that appear to indicate trends in the data that were not statistically significant.

EFFECTS AMONG THOSE WHO CLEARLY ACCEPTED MODULE SERVICE

In this section, we present findings of differences in outcomes between two groups, those receiving high and medium intensity of service, and those in the control group who were not referred to service.

We observed no significant long-term (twelve-month) differences between the total service and control study groups for any of the twelve outcomes. However, for two functional outcomes—namely, contentment and mobility—we detected statistically significant subgroup effects. For contentment we observed less deterioration among those who received module service than for controls. This effect was found in two of the eighteen subgroups (Table 7.1). At entry into the study, persons in these subgroups were younger and better off in terms of activities of daily living. When we examined the subgroup differences in mean deterioration in contentment between the service and control groups, we found a trend in the same direction which was not statistically significant. This was observed in five additional subgroups. Persons in these five subgroups included those who were better off socially, mentally, and had potentially low risk diagnoses.

In contrast to the contentment effect, a statistically significant long-term effect in mobility among certain subgroups was demonstrated as greater deterioration for those who received module service than for controls. This mobility effect was observed in three different subgroups (Table 7.1). Unlike those showing the contentment effect, people in these three subgroups included those who initially were more physically ill with potentially high risk chronic disease, and were moderately active socially. This mobility effect

Table 7.1

Percent Estimates of 12-Month Effects,
High and Medium Service Intensity vs. Controls,
By Type of Outcome and By Subgroup[1,2]

| | | Type of Outcome | |
Subgroup	ADL	Mobility	Contentment
Age			
45–64 years	——	——	+24*
65–74 years	−12	−26	——
75 years and older	——	——	——
Social Class (Hollingshead)			
Classes I–IV	——	——	+16
Class V	−13	——	——
Social Role and Activities			
Much involvement	——	——	+20
Moderate involvement	——	−17*	——
Uninvolved	——	——	——
Social Desolation			
No personal loss events	——	——	+16
1–4 personal loss events	——	−24	——
Primary Diagnosis			
Low risk	——	——	——
High risk	−12	−24*	——
ADL			
0–2 dependency	−11	——	+18*
3–6 dependency	——	——	——
Severity of Illness			
0–2 + low risk	——	——	+21
0–2 + high risk	−21	−23*	——
Orientation (MSQ)			
8–10 correct answers	——	−22	+11
0–7 correct answers	——	——	——

1 Each number in this table represents the difference between (1) the percent who showed a specific outcome among those in the service study group and (2) the percent who showed the same outcome among those not referred to the program. For example, in Table 7.1, the estimate of 24% for the outcome on contentment in the subgroup 45–64 years was derived as follows: 31% of those who received module service and 55% of controls deteriorated in contentment; thus 55% minus 31% is 24%—the estimate of relationship or beneficial effect attributed to service.

2 Subgroups and outcomes are described in Figure 7.1.

* An asterisk following a number indicates a statistically significant finding using X^2 with $p \leq .05$; numbers without asterisks have been added to show trends in the data which were not statistically significant.

− A "minus" preceding a number indicates greater deterioration or frequency in the service group.

+ A "plus" preceding a number indicates greater deterioration or frequency in the control group.

was observed in three other subgroups although these findings were not statistically significant. Persons in the latter subgroups included those who were older, had experienced personal losses, and were mentally oriented.

No statistically significant sub-group differences were observed in the remaining ten outcomes of ADL, walking, disability days, mortality, mental orientation, observation and clear thinking, economic dependence, social role and activities, admission to acute care facility and admission to extended care facility.

We found a trend in ADL that was not statistically significant (Table 7.1). In five subgroups, deterioration in ADL was found to be greater for those who received module service than for controls. This included persons in separate subgroups who were initially older, either moderately or not severely ill, had a potentially high risk chronic disease, and were lowest in social position.

We did not observe significant differences between the total service and control group in any outcome at six months. A statistically significant six-month effect was found in certain subgroups for one outcome, observation and clear thinking (Table 7.2). These were transient effects and did not appear as twelve-month effects. In this case, controls deteriorated less than those who recieved module service. Our analysis showed this effect in four subgroups. Also, a significant difference in one subgroup was observed in number of admissions to an acute care facility.

The significant findings presented in Tables 7.1 and 7.2 are concentrated in a few columns. It should be noted that when a statistically significant difference was detected in a specific homogeneous subgroup, it appeared in only one category within that subgroup. This suggests an artifact in the data which may be due to some correlation between the various subgroups. For example, taking the mobility column in Table 7.1, the persons in each of three subgroups may have tended to have potentially high risk chronic diseases and may have been more severely ill. Thus, it would not be distinctly different groups of persons with significant findings but, possibly, a group of persons with characteristics that were commonly shared. The extent to which this hypothesis is supported has not been determined. These same observations generally apply to the data presented in Tables 7.3 and 7.4.

Table 7.2

Percent Estimates of 6 Month Effects,
High and Medium Service Intensity vs. Controls,
By Type of Outcome and By Subgroup[1,2]

| Subgroup | Type of Outcome | | | |
	Observation and Clear Thinking	Social Role and Activities	Admission to Acute Care Facility	Admission to Extended Care Facility
Age				
45–64 years	——	——	——	−6
65–74 years	——	——	——	——
75 years and older	——	——	——	−13
Social Class (Hollingshead)				
Classes I–IV	−17	——	−12	——
Class V	——	−10	——	——
Social Role and Activities				
Much involvement	−32*	——	−16*	——
Moderate involvement	——	——	——	——
Uninvolved	——	——	——	——
Social Desolation				
No personal loss events	——	——	——	——
1–4 personal loss events	——	——	——	——
Primary Diagnosis				
Low risk	——	−8	——	——
High risk	−19*	——	−16	——
ADL				
0–2 dependency	−16*	——	−13	——
3–6 dependency	——	−9	——	——
Severity of Illness				
0–2 + low risk	——	——	——	——
0–2 + high risk	−24*	——	−20	——
Orientation (MSQ)				
8–10 correct answers	−13	——	−10	——
0–7 correct answers	——	−24	——	——

[1] See Footnote 1, Table 7.1.
[2] Subgroups and outcomes are described in Figure 7.1.
* An asterisk following a number indicates a statistically significant finding using X^2 with $p \leq .05$; numbers without asterisks have been added to show trends in the data which were not statistically significant.
− A "minus" preceding a number indicates greater deterioration or frequency in the service group.

Table 7.3

Percent Estimates of 12-Month Relationships, Low Service Intensity
vs. Controls, By Outcome and By Subgroup[1, 2, 3]

| | Type of Outcome | |
Subgroup	Disability Days	Orientation
Age		
45–64 years	——	——
65–74 years	——	——
75 years and older	——	——
Social Class (Hollingshead)		
Classes I–IV	——	——
Class V	——	−21*
Social Role and Activities		
Much involvement	−18*	——
Moderate involvement	——	——
Uninvolved	——	——
Social Desolation		
No personal loss events	——	——
1–4 personal loss events	——	——
Primary Diagnosis		
Low risk	——	——
High risk	−13*	——
ADL		
0–2 dependency	−11*	——
3–6 dependency	——	——
Severity of Illness		
0–2 + low risk	——	——
0–2 + high risk	−16*	——
Orientation (MSQ)		
8–10 correct answers	——	——
0–7 correct answers	——	——

[1] See Footnote 1, Table 7.1.
[2] Data are presented as estimates of relationship, not as effects of module service.
[3] Subgroups and outcomes are described in Figure 7.1.
* An asterisk following a number indicates a statistically significant finding using X^2 with $p \leq .05$; numbers without asterisks have been added to show trends in the data which were not statistically significant.
− A "minus" preceding a number indicates greater deterioration or frequency in the service group.

Table 7.4

Percent Estimates of 6-Month Relationships, Low Service Intensity
vs. Controls, By Outcome and By Subgroup[1, 2, 3]

		Type of Outcome	
Subgroup	ADL	Contentment	Orientation
Age			
45–64 years	——	+13*	——
65–74 years	——	——	——
75 years and older	——	——	——
Social Class (Hollingshead)			
Classes I–IV	——	+11*	+16*
Class V	——	——	——
Social Role and Activities			
Much involvement	——	——	+15*
Moderate involvement	——	——	——
Uninvolved	——	——	——
Social Desolation			
No personal loss events	——	——	——
1–4 personal loss events	+14	——	——
Primary Diagnosis			
Low risk	——	——	+12*
High risk	——	——	——
ADL			
0–2 dependency	——	——	+13*
3–6 dependency	−9*	——	——
Severity of Illness			
0–2 + low risk	——	——	+15*
0–2 + high risk	——	——	+13*
Orientation (MSQ)			
8–10 correct answers	——	——	+9*
0–7 correct answers	——	——	——

[1] See Footnote 1, Table 7.1.
[2] Data are presented as estimates of relationship, not as effects of module service.
[3] Subgroups and outcomes are described in Figure 7.1.
* An asterisk following a number indicates a statistically significant finding using X^2 with $p \leq .05$; numbers without asterisks have been added to show trends in the data which were not statistically significant.
− A "minus" preceding a number indicates greater deterioration or frequency in the service group.
+ A "plus" preceding a number indicates greater deterioration or frequency in the control group.

CHANGES AMONG THOSE WHO RECEIVED
MINIMAL OR NO SERVICE

As patients were not forced to accept module service, services were not always accepted; and outcomes among those who received minimal or no service (low intensity of service group) are not interpretable as effects of service. Outcomes in this group are more accurately expressed as changes or effects related to refusal or noncompliance. In Chapter 6, we stated that the essentially non-served group, in contrast to the group that followed through with module service, tended to include more men and more economically independent people. In comparison to the control group, the essentially nonserved group also included more who were independent economically. This raised the likelihood of a self-selection bias in our data, the influence of which was not analyzed, but must be taken into account when interpreting the findings of the study.

By statistical test, we did not observe either six- or twelve-month significant differences in functional changes, institutionalization, or mortality between the total control group of patients and the group that received minimal or no service. Among the eighteen homogeneous subgroups, however, some significant differences were observed. Overall, we found 15 such differences in 456 comparisons.

At twelve months (Table 7.3), four subgroups demonstrated a greater number of days of disability for low intensity service than for controls. Persons in these subgroups included those who were initially better off in ADL and those who had potentially high risk chronic diseases. As shown in Table 7.4, significant differences were noted at six months in a few homogeneous subgroups, although they were not sustained for the full year. First, some subgroups of control patients deteriorated more frequently in mental orientation than did subgroups that did not use module service. Certain control subgroups also had more frequent deterioration in contentment. The types of control patients who deteriorated more frequently in mental orientation included those who, at entry into the study, were better off physically, mentally, and socially. Control subgroups that experienced more deterioration in contentment were those that included younger patients, 45–64 years of age, and patients in the higher classes of social position.

SUMMATION

Considering the information presented in Chapter 6 and in this chapter, we observed that women were more likely to use the services of the chronic disease module than men. Also, those who were economically dependent and those receiving public assistance to pay for health care were more likely to use the service than economically independent persons. People who did not use module services tended to be men and the economically independent. In contrast to users, nonusers appeared to be more able and active, and more stable in mental orientation, satisfaction, and morale early in the study. They were comparatively young, less ill, less disabled, mentally well-oriented, socially active, and of higher social position. This pattern of use of module service, and the possible underlying social, psychological, motivational, and situational determinants, cannot be easily explained on the basis of our descriptive information. The phenomenon of acceptance and use of service by the older chronically ill population is an important area that should be further studied.

Whatever the explanatory variables may be in terms of use and non-use of module service, it was evident that a self-selection bias occurred in our study sample. Therefore, the assumption that we had randomly distributed patients into the two study groups may have been weakened. Nevertheless, those who did not use module service were followed in the study and information collected in order to give further insight into this group.

In our analysis, we found that people who refused module service and initially had potentially high risk diseases experienced greater number of days of disability during the twelve months than did similar subgroups of control patients. By the end of the full twelve months this study group did not differ significantly from the control group in any of the other outcomes under study. Thus, except for disability days, the experience of persons in each group was no different over the long-term. This was not the picture for those who used module service, as described below.

Similar to findings in the Continued Care Study, module service had specific consequences for persons with particular characteristics. Katz et al. (1972) stated that the relatively young and least disabled persons were more likely to maintain or improve function and to benefit from nursing service. Our study showed that younger persons who received module service, as well as those who were least ill and disabled, experienced higher levels of satisfaction and moral than persons who did not receive such service. Thus, it appeared that among persons who had the greater potential for improvement, those who received health assistant service were consequently better off in terms of satisfaction. For such persons, the health assistant had apparently provided enough physical and psychosocial care and support to enhance levels of satisfaction over a long period of time.

In the Continued Care Study, nursing service resulted in improved physical and mental function among those who had the most potential for improvement. For similar patients, the present study showed that health assistant service did not demonstrate statistically significant benefits in physical and mental function. Comparison of both studies provides suggestive information about the relative effect of nursing service and health assistant service with patients requiring similar levels of service intensity. Such a question is relevant and should be addressed in future studies.

Katz and his associates (1972) observed that persons who had less potential for maintenance and improvement were the ones in whom service did not show beneficial effects. This was supported in our study, where the long-term effect of module service tended toward decreased physical function in terms of mobility and activities of daily living. This occurred particularly among persons who were very old or severely ill and disabled and, thus, had less potential for maintenance and improvement of function. This outcome suggested a possible "dependency effect" of sustained service which was previously cited by Katz et al. (1972). With regard to this, future studies might address the influence of high intensity of service on dependency and its relationship to, for example, patient motivation and self-care practices.

Module service was also associated with a transient, short-term effect in the direction of decreased observation and clear thinking. This effect occurred particularly among individuals who were most severely ill and disabled, adding support to the view that those with less potential to maintain or improve their status would benefit least from service, but tend to use more services. These short-term specific consequences, again, tend to replicate the interval results reported by Katz et al. (1972).

REFERENCES

Katz, S., Ford, A. B., Downs, T. D., Adams, M., and Rusby, D. 1972. *Effects of Continued Care: A Study of Chronic Illness in the Home.* DHEW Publication No. (HSM) 73–3010. U.S. Government Printing Office, Washington, D.C., pp. 59, 62, 76–82, 93.
Feinberg, S. E. 1977. *The Analysis of Cross-Classified Categorical Data.* The MIT Press, Cambridge, Massachusetts.

Chapter 8

HEALTH CARE COSTS
RELATED TO
MODULE SERVICE

Robert Stevens
Anne Cunningham

Attention was given to the comparison of costs reported by persons who received medium and high levels of module service, as defined in Chapter 6, and by those who were not referred to module service (control group). Specifically, certain relationships between module service and use of health care resources were examined. Resources were measured in terms of dollar cost for such items as the number of days spent in a hospital or extended care facility, or the number of contacts with different types of health care personnel. In this regard, the use of four sets of resources was analyzed: acute care facilities, extended care facilities, health care personnel (including physicians, nurses, therapists, and health assistants), and all non-institutional health care resources.

Collection of cost information was through participant interviews as part of the six- and twelve-month observations of our overall study design as described in Chapter 3. The questions that were asked about resource utilization and related charges appear in Appendix B. We used regression analysis to statistically examine the interview data, with statistical controls for age, sex, and module geographic location. Two such analyses were carried out. The first analysis compared all persons referred to service with all those not referred to service. In the second analysis, those referred to service who accepted and received medium and high levels of service were compared to the control group. This second analysis, therefore, involved comparison of a group of self-selected persons, which should be kept in mind in interpreting results. A finding was considered significant when a test of statistical significance resulted in a probability level of .05 or less.

EFFECTS ON RESOURCE USE

Two opposite effects on resource use were considered possible as a result of providing module service to people in their homes. One effect could be higher health care resource use. This would occur if barriers to needed services were removed by module service. An opposite effect could occur if access to institutional care is no problem. In this case, for example, earlier discharge from an acute care hospital could occur if care in the home was available through module service. Further, a reduction in institutionalization in long-term care settings could be achieved through the provision of maintenance and support services by regular visits in the home. Such effects could occur at the same time. In general, if savings in the use of other health care resources was greater than the cost of module service, we could infer that the cost of health care for chronic disease patients could be reduced. In view of the foregoing, the results of our cost studies are reported below under each of three resource categories.

    1. Cost of Institutionalization

        a. Acute care facility use

           The analysis of responses showed that for all participants there was no statistically significant overall effect of module service on the use of acute care facilities (Table 8.1). For persons receiving medium and high levels of

Table 8.1

The Use and Cost of Health Institutions
For Service and Control Groups

	Observed Average			Comparisons Between Control and Group Referred to Service[a]		Comparisons Between Control and Group Referred to Service with Medium and High Levels of Service[a]	
	Group Not Referred to Service	Group Referred to Service	Group Referred to Service with Medium and High Levels of Service	Estimated Difference	Significance Level	Estimated Difference	Significance Level[b]
1) Days in Acute Care Facility							
First 6 months	7.0	7.4	8.9	.29	.78	1.9	.17
Second 6 months	4.6	4.9	4.9	.27	.81	0.3	.83
2) Days in Extended Care Facility							
First 6 months	6.1	3.4	3.6	−2.4	.15	−1.4	.54
Second 6 months	8.4	4.9	8.9	−3.5	.29	1.7	.66
3) Cost of institutionalization ($)							
Sixth month	129	72	75	−63	.04*	−51	.21
Twelfth month	69	90	51	28	.43	−23	.62

* Statistically significant at .05 level
[a] Regression estimates. Significance level is based on the F test.
[b] Caution is needed in interpreting these results as those with medium and high levels of service were not randomly chosen from among those referred to service.

service, an increased use of acute care was observed during the first six months but not in the following six months. The data showed a decline in the use of acute care facilities for all study participants following the first six-month period.

b. Extended care facility use
There was no statistically significant overall effect of module service on the use of extended care facilities (Table 8.1). However, regression analysis estimated a reduction of 2.4 days of extended care facility use in the first six-month period for those referred to module service. This finding represented more than a one-third reduction in nursing home use by persons referred to module service. Average use of extended care facilities increased by about one-third for all groups between the first and second six-month period. In addition to the data reported in Table 8.1, a result of particular interest was that the low intensity service group also had the lowest estimated use of extended care facilities in both time periods.

c. Combined use of facilities
A measure of the combined use of acute and extended care facilities was obtained. From our interview data we computed average costs incurred by the participants for the thirty-day period coiniding with the sixth and twelfth month after the person entered the study. The results, as reported in Table 8.2, indicated that during the sixth month the group referred to module service incurred about one-half the cost for institutional care incurred by the control group, a sixty dollar difference. This difference was statistically significant. Also, those referred to service who received medium and high levels of module service were estimated to have incurred the same lower level of institutional cost.

In the twelfth month after the person's entry into the study, the observed results were not statistically different. While the observed average cost of institutionalization among those not referred to service declined from $129 to $62, the cost for the total group offered module service increased from $72 to $90. However, those receiving medium and high levels of module service averaged the lowest costs, decreasing from $75 to $51.

Table 8.2

Physician Contacts and the Cost of Physician Services
For Service and Control Groups

	Observed Average			Comparisons Between Control and Group Referred to Service[a]		Comparisons Between Control and Group Referred to Service with Medium and High Levels of Service[a]	
	Group Not Referred to Service	Group Referred to Service	Group Referred to Service with Medium and High Levels of Service	Estimated Difference	Significance Level	Estimated Difference	Significance Level[b]
Number of contacts with physicians							
Sixth month	2.3	1.5	1.7	−.83	.02*	−.28	.53
Twelfth month	1.2	1.4	1.1	.28	.38	−.02	.96
Cost of physician services ($)							
Sixth month	33	26	22	−9.1	.25	−13	.22
Twelfth month	20	30	25	12.2	.26	7	.62

* Statistically significant at .05 level
a Regresson estimates. Significance level is based on the F test.
b Caution is needed in interpreting these results as those with medium and high levels of service were not randomly chosen from among those referred to service.

2. Cost of Health Care Personnel

    a. Use of physicians and other doctors

    Table 8.2 shows that in the sixth month persons re-
    ferred to module service averaged about one-third less
    contacts with physicians than those not referred. The
    observed difference of 1.5 as compared to 2.3 contacts
    was statistically significant. In the twelfth month, differ-
    ences between the groups in number of physician con-
    tacts were not statistically significant.

    The cost per month of the participants' use of all
    physicians and other types of doctors (e.g. psychologists,
    dentists, ophthalmologists, podiatrists) was examined
    through the interview data. In the sixth month after enter-
    ing the study, those participants offered service had
    appreciably smaller average costs in this category, $26
    as compared to $33 for the control group. For those
    receiving medium or high levels of module service, the
    average cost was still lower, $22. However, for the
    twelfth month, those offered service appeared to have
    average payments for physician services that were about
    $12 higher than those not referred to module service, but
    this difference was not statistically significant.

    b. Use of nurses

    Reported contacts with registered nurses and licensed
    practical nurses during the sixth and twelfth month of
    participation in the study were not significantly different
    for those offered and not offered service (Table 8.3).
    However, over the first six months, persons who received
    medium or high intensity of service reported 2.2 more
    contacts per month with nurses than did persons in the
    control group, a statistically significant difference.

    c. Use of other health care providers

    This category included contacts with all other health
    care providers (excluding doctors and nurses). Records
    kept by module health assistants indicated that there was
    an average of 3.2 visits per month to the group receiving
    medium and high levels of module service. The number of
    contacts with all other health providers reported by this
    group in the sixth month after study entry was 4.3 (Table
    8.3) and therefore is consistent with module visit records.
    This finding was statistically significant. In the twelfth

Table 8.3

The Number of Contacts with Nurses and Other Health Care Providers, and Total Non-Institutional Health Care Costs for Service and Control Groups

	Observed Average			Comparisons Between Control and Group Referred to Service[a]		Comparisons Between Control and Group Referred to Service with Medium and High Levels of Service[a]	
	Group Not Referred to Service	Group Referred to Service	Group Referred to Service with Medium and High Levels of Service	Estimated Difference	Significance Level	Estimated Difference	Significance Level[b]
Number of Contacts With Nurses[c]							
Sixth month	1.5	1.7	3.2	.16	.85	2.2	.05*[b]
Twelfth month	1.6	4.0	3.8	2.2	.31	1.1	.69
Number of Contacts With Other Health Care Providers							
Sixth month	1.8	3.0	5.9	1.1	.21	4.3	.00*[b]
Twelfth month	1.9	5.0	4.6	2.9	.19	1.4	.61
Total Non-Institutional Health Care Costs ($)							
Sixth month	66	76	74	8.0	.57	-6.4	.75
Twelfth month	59	78	80	20.5	.21	17.8	.39

* Statistically significant at .05 level
[a] Regression estimates. Significance level is based on the F test.
[b] Caution is needed in interpreting these results as those with medium and high levels of service were not randomly chosen from among those referred to service.
[c] Registered nurses and licensed practical nurses.

month of service, a lower number of contacts with all other health care providers was estimated for persons offered service at the medium and high levels of intensity of service, but the differences were not significant.

3. Cost of Non-Institutional Health Care Resource Use

This category included health care providers, medications, and other related costs.

Non-institutional costs for those referred to module service tended to be somewhat greater than for those not referred to module service. These differences were not statistically significant, however. In the twelfth month, there appeared to be an increase of about $20 per month in non-institutional health care costs for those offered service. This difference was not statistically significant.

SUMMATION

Several cost parameters were measured in interviews at the sixth and twelfth month of the study. These parameters included use of acute and extended care facilities, use of health care personnel, and costs of institutional and noninstitutional health care, considered separately. Two comparisons were made for each selected parameter. The first was a comparison of differences between all those referred to service and all those not referred (controls). The second comparison was between those persons who received medium and high levels of service and the control group. The latter comparison was more indicative of effects of module service on resource use for cost-estimation purposes, while the former was more appropriate for statistical tests of group differences.

The only comparisons with significant differences were observed at the sixth-month interview. The costs of institutionalization in the prior one-month period were lower for persons referred to service than for controls. Another finding was that the number of contacts with doctors in the prior one-month period was greater for the control group. These results suggested an intermediate (six month) effect of module service on reducing health care costs.

In addition to these results, several trends were suggested by the data. At the time of the sixth-month interview, persons in the control group showed higher utilization of extended care facilities for the prior six-month period than either all persons referred to service or the self-selected group that received medium and high levels of service. These differences between groups were significant at the .20 level but not at the .05 level of significance. Perhaps, due to increased extended care facility use, noninstitutional health care costs were lower for the prior one-month period at the sixth-month interview for those not referred to service than for those who received service.

The results of the cost studies of resources indicate: (1) a moderate impact of module service on reducing health care costs within the first six months of the service period; (2) that the reduction in costs incurred by those receiving module service was approximately balanced by the modest cost of module service; and (3) that some types of home care for certain categories of patients could significantly reduce the costs of caring for chronic disease patients.

Chapter 9

POLICY IMPLICATIONS

Joseph Papsidero
Sidney Katz

The findings of our research provide a basis for analyzing legislation and related regulations intended to facilitate access to and appropriate use of home care. Given a description of the intent of legislation, it is possible to critique regulations in the light of our research findings, and then identify certain implications for improved policy directions in long-term care. This applies, in particular, to Medicare and Medicaid financing of home care. Of equal relevance, are implications for quality assurance through the Professional Standards Review Organization (PSRO) program. The focus of such policy analysis is the need for more appropriate entry to care and better cost-effectiveness.

With regard to the Medicare and Medicaid approach to financing, we must direct attention to the individual's entry into care and its discontinuance as determinants of the limits of payments. Quality assurance must be critiqued in terms of the structural and decision-making capabilities for entry and disposition, as well as the criteria that can be used to determine the capacity of service programs to achieve socially relevant objectives.

The foregoing describes a policy analysis view that is used in the remainder of this chapter.

MEDICARE AND MEDICAID

The hospital insurance benefits of Medicare (Part A) provide payment for home care for persons who are confined at home because of a problem of mobility or function. Payment is not provided for problems that do not involve health status, such as lack of transportation. Physicians or nurses must attest to the need for home care based on a mobility or functional problem. Home care benefits are available for a single episode of illness only, after a stay of at least three days in a hospital or skilled nursing home. Within fourteen days after discharge from the institution, a plan of care must be filed; and the patient must be under the care of a physician. A maximum of 100 visits is provided per year, and there is no financial means test.

The regulations permit payment for physician services, skilled nursing, physical therapy, and speech therapy on an intermittent basis. The definition of skilled nursing services includes administering medications and providing instruction for self-administered procedures, as in diabetic care. Such instruction may be given by a registered nurse or licensed practical nurse to the family or patient. Service from a home health aide is limited to part-time personal care and is reimbursed only if skilled nursing care is needed and delivered at the same time by a certified home health agency.

In contrast to Medicare, which was designed to finance limited medical coverage for the aged, the intent of Medicaid was to provide broad health care financing for the poor. Eligibility for public assistance establishes eligibility for medical assistance that is reimbursed by public funds. In addition to persons who are economically needy, those with high medical expenses are eligible for Medicaid assistance if they are defined as medically needy. Determination of the scope and size of the program is left to each state, although participating states must reimburse for seven basic services: inpatient hospital care; outpatient hospital care; laboratory and x-ray services; skilled nursing home care; physician services; and early periodic screening, diagnosis, and treatment for children less than twenty-one years old. In addition, an unlimited number of services can be reimbursed at state option with federal matching funds, including such services as physical therapy and preventive and rehabilitative services. Home health services are included for anyone entitled to skilled nursing home services, and eligibility follows the same general pattern as that defined by the regulations for Medicare.

Medicare and Medicaid regulations define eligibility in terms of age and economic criteria. Decisions about entry into care and about the types of services needed are made by physicians and nurses, generally in institutions. Since requirements concerning professional practice and the processes of care are minimal, criteria are interpreted flexibly with a significant aim to achieve government reimbursement for services. As a result, professionals define entry into care and then allocate their services, a situation that can lead to uncontrolled marketing of such services. Better specification of the entry, service, and exit criteria would improve the rational use of Medicare and Medicaid financing. In this regard, it is our premise that current criteria do not implement the Medicare and Medicaid legislative intent to finance necessary services that are beneficial. In particular, criteria that reflect available information about impact of long-term care are not visible. Such information is provided by the Chronic Disease Module study reported in this book and by our previous experiments and longitudinal studies.

In the Continued Care Study, relatively young (fifty to sixty-four years), less disabled, and less severely ill persons were more likely to benefit in physical and mental function after receiving long-term visiting nurse services than were similar people in a control group who did not receive such services (Katz et al. 1972). Admissions to nursing homes were also delayed among people who received visiting nurse services. In contrast, the presence of visiting nurse services was associated with an increased use of hospitals and professionals among the oldest, very disabled, and severely ill people when compared to similar controls. Despite an increased use of services, the high risk group (older, very disabled, and severely ill) did not benefit in physical and mental function from the visiting nurse program. In the Chronic Disease Module study reported here, the relatively young, less disabled, and less severely ill experienced higher levels of satisfaction and morale after receiving home services by a health assistant than did similar people in a control group who did not receive such services. Avoidance of functional deterioration was not demonstrated as an effect of home care by health assistants. In both experiments, consequences appear to be specific with respect to the type of treatment and type of patient. Where benefits were associated with home care services, such benefits accrued to patients with the most potential for improvement—as, for example, the younger and less disabled.

As complementing information, ten-year follow-up studies of patients with hip fracture and stroke revealed that the likelihood of recovery decreased over time in the presence of sophisticated rehabilitation therapy (Katz et al. 1966, 1967). The likelihood of recovery of function virtually disappeared eighteen to twenty-four months after the onset of disability, if such function had not returned by that time. This information has implications for the definition of criteria with regard to the duration of delivery and financing of technology-rich rehabilitation services.

Our experiences with longitudinal studies of disabled people also led us to consider that service goals shift over time after the onset of disability. Use of technology-rich medical and rehabilitative services to effect improvement is appropriate for about a year, at the most two years after onset. Thereafter, service goals are more appropriately defined as maintenance of function, support of social needs, and provision of access to more sophisticated services at times of increased need. This implies that long-term services for people with less potential for improvement should be organized with more emphasis on planning, teaching, monitoring, support, and coordination than on diagnosis, medical treatment, and consultation. The issue to be resolved in this regard is one of appropriate changes in the balance between supportive services and technology-rich services over time.

Based on our research experiences, we recommend that three categories of care be recognized within regulations that deal with the financing of long-term care services. The three categories of services should be distinguished as those that aim, respectively, toward (1) full or partial recovery of function in organized programs that include skilled provider technology, (2) maintenance and support through means other than skilled technology, and (3) support in anticipation of death with dignity. Criteria for eligibility, entry, and exit should vary for the three categories of services, as should accountability. A separate coordinating activity should be responsible for the appropriate movement of patients between different parts of the system and for making services of each category available in the other areas when needed. The coordinating activity should have its own criteria and accountability.

With regard to criteria for eligibility, research experiences such as those described here provide guiding principles about the types of goals that are likely to be achieved by different categories of service programs and about the types of people who are likely to respond to each form of service. For example, our studies indicate that we can identify aged people with recent onset of disability (e.g., fracture of the hip, rheumatoid arthritis, etc.) who are likely to benefit from the comprehensive services of rehabilitation hospitals or specialized outpatient programs (Katz et al. 1963, 1968.) We have also shown that, following the initial intensive technology-rich services, patients with these conditions who do not have other severe complicating factors such as poor mental function or major disease are likely to improve function under the continuing long-term care of skilled visiting nurses (Katz 1972). Upon the achievement of a sustained period of improvement, such skilled services can be discontinued. If no improvement is observed for about eighteen months, further skilled services are not likely to benefit, and supportive services other than skilled technology are needed. Current information does not support the financing of a high intensity of technology-rich services in all of the foregoing circumstances. For example, a requirement that physicians should visit patients in nursing homes every thirty days is not a logical generalization. In view of available knowledge about the potential consequences of services for specific types of patients, use of non-institutional skilled care alternatives and trained health assistants should achieve a more rational balance among cost, effectiveness, and satisfaction.

Those who decide about eligibility for long-term care, its intensity, and its change or discontinuance should be knowledgeable about the potential effectiveness or lack of effectiveness of specific services for specific types of patients. They should know the circumstances that foster unnecessary dependency. They should also know the relative effects and costs of alternative means of care. Unfortunately, it is our experience that the qualifications of those who currently make decisions are limited in these aspects. Hospital providers often have little specific knowledge and experience about the impact of rehabilitation and nursing care for the disabled, much less about the relative impact and cost of alternative modes of long-term care. Yet, these providers define entry and intensity. Current regulations assign responsibility for decisions about eligibility to professions and organizations without due concern for their qualifications to make appropriate decisions. In the presence of limited qualifications, their decisions are based on the limited capabilities of patients, rather than on the recognized potential of patients and the potential of service programs. It is no wonder that the decision is generally made to refer to services within the control of the decision-maker's profession or organization, without primary concern for outcome and cost-effectiveness. Discharge planning in hospitals is generally not sophisticated, and providers in nursing homes rarely even consider it. Coordination of services is implemented infrequently. In the presence of institutional and professional orientations, the patient's potential is secondary and only vaguely addressed. Costly, improper placement occurs all too often. Certification of agencies or individuals to provide long-term care and to make decisions about eligibility or referral should be based on demonstrated knowledge about the potential consequences of long-term services for specific types of patients, as well as about the relative effects and relative costs of alternative means of care. The fact that long-term care comprises a large part of the care given by nurses and physicians indicates that examinations for licensing of these professionals should include the testing of the relevant knowledge from this and our other studies. Certification of agencies for discharge planning, coordination, and long-term services should, with increased emphasis, evaluate and attest to the required competencies and knowledges. From the viewpoint of cost-effective long-term care, we do not currently meet even minimum requirements for licensing professionals and certification of agencies and institutions.

QUALITY ASSURANCE AND LONG-TERM CARE

Quality of care is regarded as a multidimensional concept having different definitions. Consumers, nurses, physicians, administrators, third party payors, and legislators hold different views of what constitutes quality. Most define quality in terms of either the process, the outcome, or the structure of care. Some emphasize that more care is not necessarily better, and that cost is integral to quality.

In recent years, we have experienced the development of formal mechanisms to assure that people receive high quality care. These mechanisms are called quality assurance systems. Forces that influenced this development include the emerging view of health care as a social right, an increase in consumer sophistication, the recognition that health care is a limited national resource, and the need that costs be controlled.

A quality assurance system is the complete system for reviewing and making judgments about quality of care and taking action to improve it. The opportunity to implement quality assurance broadly was provided by the Social Security Amendments of 1972. Specifically, Public Law 92-603, HR-1 authorized the Secretary of the Department of Health, Education, and Welfare to establish Professional Standards Review Organizations (PSRO's) to review health care provided under Medicare, Medicaid, and Maternal and Child Health programs. PSRO's are required to review institutional care, including short-stay general hospitals, tuberculosis hospitals, mental health hospitals, and, in time, skilled nursing facilities and intermediate care facilities. Eventually, PSRO's will be required to review noninstitutional care, although such review is now possible upon request and if the Secretary of the Department of Health, Education, and Welfare approves.

Recent PSRO guidelines for the review of long-term care emphasize medical necessity, appropriateness of admission, continued stay review, and medical care evaluation studies. The guidelines recognize the importance of different types of providers, and require involvement of a multidisciplinary group. In order to certify necessity and appropriateness of admission, the guidelines require pre-admission certification either by a hospital review staff or by an approved independent organization. Other requirements include concurrent quality review to determine necessity of continued stay and appropriateness of services provided. Medical record review, at least one bedside review per year, and medical care evaluation studies are also specified.

We cannot overemphasize the consideration that quality assurance in long-term care must recognize unique characteristics and care requirements of the aged and chronically ill. Aged people with chronic conditions differ from people with acute episodes of disease. For example, the elderly with chronic conditions are more likely to have multiple problems which draw concurrently on multiple services. Home-making, medical, and income services are more likely to be required for long periods of time. In the absence of cure, outcome goals are more often formulated in such terms as restoration of function to the best possible level and maintenance at that level. Long-term care must, thus, provide prolonged and coordinated multidisciplinary rehabilitation services that depend on uniquely integrated management and record systems. Rather than primary prevention, secondary prevention and slowing of deterioration become the explicit preventive goals of service providers. In this context, successful providers must have different motivations and incentives. Relatedly, patients and their families must change their expectations from those of cure to those of coping.

In contrast to acute care, the long-term care patient's entry into an institution or contact with a physician does not generally mean that full care will be provided in one place. For such patients, a community orientation to long-term care is essential. However, our current organization and delivery of care generally favors an episodic approach that tends to satisfy mainly diagnostic and acute care needs, while only partially satisfying chronic disease and long-term care needs. A new approach for long-term care of the chronically ill and aged is a definite need. An examination of the unique characteristics of long-term care will help to define this need for changes in the system.

Long-term care includes institutional and noninstitutional services for people with chronic conditions. Such conditions are recurrent or persistent deviations from normal health which may be experienced as symptoms, illnesses, handicaps, disabilities, or impairments. Decreased function and shorter life span are usual consequences, and the associated outcome of increased dependence has serious affects. The continuing cost of care greatly diminishes socioeconomic productivity.

The needs and demands associated with chronic conditions are generally expressed in physical, psychological, social, and environmental terms. Long-term care activities bear upon such needs and demands to achieve improved outcomes at certain costs. Within this framework, service decisions are required which improve our effectiveness in health maintenance, illness intervention, and the quality of life. These decisions must also be socially responsible in that they satisfy concerns for available, accessible, and efficient services. In long-term care, service systems are needed that integrate basic living supports and multidisciplinary elements whereby continuous services are provided over long periods of time in a dignified and socially responsible manner. Even as we stress continuity, we must avoid inappropriate dependence and discontinue unnecessary services. In view of the uniqueness of long-term care, the implications for quality assurance become clear.

Quality assurance should address itself to programs of care and their capacity to achieve objectives in relation to socially relevant goals. Socially relevant goals are to restore and maintain the maximal level of full or partial independence in function, restore and maintain stability of the medical condition, maintain maximal dignity when the patient's condition is deteriorating, and return the patient home whenever possible. In long-term care, the foregoing goals may be assigned to three types of programs and objectives as described below.

Rehabilitation hospitals, chronic disease hospitals and other technology-rich institutional programs provide special diagnostic, therapeutic, and rehabilitation services that aim to restore full or partial function of the patient and stabilize medical conditions that are not under control. For patients who need the services provided by such institutions, the objectives related to these goals are as follows: (1) improve function, stabilize medical status, and return home; (2) improve function, stabilize medical status, and return home after temporary referral to a nursing home; (3) improve function, stabilize medical status, and transfer to a nursing home or related institution for long-term support not available at home and in the community; (4) provide specialized supports for the patient who is deteriorating rapidly in function or is medically at risk and not expected to recover.

Nursing homes or related types of institutions primarily provide basic living services for prolonged periods of time, including regularly needed care for medically stable conditions. For those in nursing homes or related types of institutions, the objectives are: (1) improve or maintain function, provide temporary functional and medical supports that do not require technology-rich institutional resources, and return patient home; (2) maintain partial self-functioning capabilities and provide long-term basic living services and medical care that are not available to the dependent patient at home; (3) support the patient who is deteriorating slowly, who does not need the resources of a technology-rich institution, and for whom necessary supports are not available at home.

Care in the home or a related type of noninstitutional setting is the third type of program, and related objectives are: (1) improve function to full independence in order to enable the individual to remain at home and care for self; (2) improve or maintain function and enable the individual to remain at home with family or community support; (3) enable the deteriorating person to remain at home as long as possible, when improvement and maintenance are no longer possible.

The foregoing has significant implications for both the assessment methods and criteria that are included in systems for long-term care quality assurance. The unique characteristics and care requirements that we describe indicate the need for special types of assessments. Since improvement and maintenance of function are of primary importance among the goals of long-term care, the classes of problems to be reviewed must encompass function in addition to the diagnostic classes usually reviewed in acute care. Outcome criteria must reflect the dimensions of potential for change and the availability of family and community support, since the types of services to which patients should be referred are critically dependent on these factors. Relatedly, criteria are needed for both entry and disposition. In addition to criteria for short-term outcomes, criteria for long-term outcomes need to be established. Finally, structural criteria take on special meaning in view of the importance of co-ordinated, multiple institutional and noninstitutional services at given points in time and serially over time. The presently reported study and our previously reported research experiences contribute specific knowledge that is useful in developing quality assurance systems for long-term care.

The assessment schedule described in Chapter 3 is an example of the assessment approach that is needed in long-term care quality assurance systems. It is derived from tested instruments and encom-passes objective and reliable measures of function that have demon-strated use in describing improvement and deterioration of patients. The assessment schedule recognizes the unique characteristics and care requirements of the aged and chronically ill. It comprehen-sively evaluates physical, psychological, social, and economic needs. It has been constructed to reflect current advanced knowledge about reliable and meaningful measures of need and multidimensional function. When used to reassess a patient at several points in time, it is sensitive to changes in the patient's health status. Detailed in-formation collected through the instrument is useful in helping to set individualized goals for care and in redefining goals iteratively on the basis of defined functional responses of the patients. Aggre-gated information about patients in long-term care programs is useful for service program evaluation, for management, and for policy-making and planning. It can serve as an evaluation for pre-admission certification to identify patient needs, to define rehabili-tation and support goals, and to establish recommendations for appropriate referral. The schedule can be used to evaluate the need for continued stay. When linked to information about the process of care, it can be used to evaluate the appropriateness of health services provided.

Information obtained through the schedule can be the basis for selecting cases for quality review, including medical care evaluation studies. Since dysfunction and lack of available social support are among the primary reasons for admitting patients to long-term care programs, cases can be selected for review on the basis of relevant functional and/or support issues, rather than on the basis of diag-nosis alone. It is more relevant in long-term care to identify cases for review as, for example, "a person with stroke who lives alone and needs assistance in bathing, dressing, and toileting," rather than merely as "a person with stroke." Similarly, it is more relevant to identify a person as having "problems of fracture of the hip, inability to ambulate without personal assistance, and confusion," rather than merely as having "fracture of the hip." Since the schedule provides for systematic evaluation in functional and support terms, cases can be selected for review in terms of classes that include function in addition to the diagnostic classes usually reviewed in acute care. We have previously described and applied profiled methods for classifying disease and disability, as well as severity of illness (Katz et al. 1972; Akpom et al. 1973).

The section on *Medicare and Medicaid* in this chapter described examples of outcomes of service programs that we observed in experimental studies. Such outcomes help to define outcome criteria for quality assurance systems. Our longitudinal studies have also contributed information about the chance for change that is useful in developing outcome criteria. In a study, for example, of patients with fracture of the hip, we found that most full and partial recoveries in walking occurred within twelve to eighteen months after fracture, and there was little likelihood of recovery after two years (Katz 1967). In that study, recovery in activities of daily living tended to precede recovery in walking, and functional recovery was generally sustained for two years or longer. Advanced age and preference disability were predictors of poor outcome. In a related study of patients with stroke, we developed similar predictive information that is useful to providers as they set appropriate goals for long-term care (Katz 1966). Such predictive information is also useful in establishing outcome criteria that retrospectively identify patients who do not respond as well as expected (i.e., deviations from the standard or expected outcome). Through in-depth record audit of these exceptions, we can discover the reasons for the lack of response, and, then, improve our approach to care.

As indicated previously, long-term care requires coordinated services at a given point in time and serially over time. It requires a community orientation, and continuity. Structural elements of organization and process must be evaluated in quality assurance systems for long-term care. Criteria are needed to evaluate the processes of admission, referral, and disposition. Congruence should be established between appropriate goals such as were defined earlier and the care program's demonstrated record with regard to admission, referral, and disposition. The capability of those who make such decisions should be evaluted with regard to their knowledge about the potential effectiveness or lack of effectiveness of specific services for specific types of patients, as well as about the relative effects and costs of alternative modes of care. The sufficiency of transfer agreements, sharing of information, and extent of functional links to the community's long-term care services must be evaluated. The experimental and longitudinal research information that have been cited here is directly useful in criteria development for evaluating these structural elements of organization and process.

SUMMATION

These research findings have implications for improved policy directions in long term care as related to financing and quality assurance. In this regard, the need to improve decisions in long-term care through better criteria for entry to care, services provided, and discontinuance of care is emphasized. We further emphasize that, in contrast to what now exists, criteria for entry, service, and discontinuance must adequately reflect what is known about the impact of long-term care. We propose that the findings of our current and previously reported longitudinal studies provide the kind of impact information upon which improved criteria can be developed. On the basis of our research findings we introduce a new framework for considering financing and decision-making. As a response to fragmented service and reflecting a systems view, our framework includes three categories of services aimed at (1) full or partial recovery of patient function in organized programs using skilled provider technology, (2) maintenance and support through means other than skilled technology, and (3) support in anticipation of death with dignity. In relation to these three categories of service, we introduce a view of coordination of services which we define as a separate coordinating activity for the movement of patients within the system, having its own criteria and its own accountability. Relatedly, we present an improved clarification of the types of goals that are likely to be achieved by the different categories of programs. We then propose that those who decide about entry, intensity, and termination of care should know about potential effectiveness of specific services for specific types of patients, the circumstances that foster dependency, and the relative effects and costs of alternative means of care. Such knowledge should be a part of their professional qualifications, which is not now the case. With regard to this, the need for change in evaluation approaches leading to certification of agencies and institutions and leading to the licensing of professionals is emphasized. In addition, we propose that quality assurance address itself to programs of care and their capacity to achieve objectives in relation to socially relevant goals unique to long-term care. Three types of programs—technology-rich institutions, nursing homes, and care in the home—are identified and the kinds of goal-oriented objectives appropriate for each are introduced. We then identify and provide examples of assessment methods we have applied to accumulate information and describe their relevance to long-term care quality assurance purposes. Then, we describe how the kinds of information obtained in our research experience can be translated into criteria for long-term care quality assurance. Such information is important in identifying more clearly the chance for change which must guide efforts to develop criteria, revise policy, improve decisions, and evaluate programs and systems of care.

REFERENCES

Akpom, C. A., Katz, S., and Densen, P. M. 1973. Methods of classifying disability and severity of illness in ambulatory care patients. *Medical Care* (Supplement) 11:125–131.
Katz, S., Ford, A. B., Moskowitz, R. W., Jackson, B. A., and Jaffe, M. W. 1963. Studies of illness in the aged: The Index of ADL: A standardized measure of biological and psycho-social function. *JAMA* 185:914–919.

Katz, S., Ford, A. B., Chinn, A. B., and Newill, V. A. 1966. Prognosis after stroke—Part II. Long-term course of 159 patients. *Medicine* 45:236–246.
Katz, S., Heiple, K. G., Downs, T. D., Ford, A. B., and Scott, C. P. 1967. Long term course of 147 patients with fracture of the hip. *Surgery, Gynecology and Obstetrics* 124:1219–1230.
Katz, S., Vignos, P. J., Jr., Moskowitz, R. W., Thompson, H. M., and Svec, K. 1968. Comprehensive outpatient care in rheumatoid arthritis, a controlled study. *JAMA* 206:1249–1254.
Katz, S., Ford, A. B., Downs, T. D., Adams, M., and Rusby, D. 1972. *Effects of Continued Care: A Study of Chronic Illness in the Home.* DHEW Publication No. (HSM) 73–3010. U.S. Government Printing Office, Washington, D.C.

Appendix A

FIRST STAGE
SCREENING FORM

SECOND STAGE
SCREENING FORM

FIRST STAGE SCREENING FORM

NURSE-PATIENT APPRAISAL AND CONTINUING CARE MODULE SCREENING QUESTIONNAIRE

1a. During the past two weeks, did the patient cut down on the things he usually does because of sickness, injury or other health problem?

yes_____ no_____

b. Was the sickness, injury or other health problem noticed more than three months ago?

yes_____ no_____

c. Is it probable that the patient's present sickness, injury or other health problem will eventuate in his cutting down on the things he usually does for at least three more months time?

yes_____ no_____

2a. During the past two weeks, did someone help the patient perform his usual activities or function because of sickness, injury or other health problem?

yes_____ no_____

b. Was the sickness, injury or other health problem noticed more than three months ago?

yes_____ no_____

c. Is it probable that the patient's present sickness, injury or other health problem will eventuate in his needing help in performing usual activities or functions for at least three months time?

yes_____ no_____

3a. During the past two weeks, did the patient require human assistance in performing the following functions because of sickness, injury or other health problem?

1. Bathing yes_____ no_____

2. Dressing yes_____ no_____

3. Walking yes_____ no_____

b. Was the sickness, injury or other health problem noticed more than three months ago?

yes_____ no_____

c. Is it probable that the patient's present sickness, injury or other
    health problem will eventuate in a need for assistance in perform-
    ing any of these functions, in his home, for at least three months
    time?

    1. Bathing   yes_____   no_____

    2. Dressing   yes_____   no_____

    3. Walking   yes_____   no_____

4a. During the past two weeks, did the patient have shortness of breath
     under any or all of the following circumstances:

    1. While performing usual
        activities?   yes_____   no_____

    2. When excited, emotionally
        upset or hurrying?   yes_____   no_____

    3. While climbing at least one
        flight of stairs or on walking
        one or two blocks?   yes_____   no_____

b. Was the shortness of breath noticed more than three months ago?

                    yes_____   no_____

c. Has the patient had persistent cough, wheezing or phlegm (sputum)
    at least daily for six months or longer?

                    yes_____   no_____

5a. During the past two weeks, did the patient have pain, swelling or
     stiffness in one or more joints?

                    yes_____   no_____

b. Was the pain, swelling or stiffness noticed more than three months
    ago?

                    yes_____   no_____

SECOND-STAGE SCREENING QUESTIONNAIRE

Answer *Either* Question 1 Or All Parts Of Question 2 And Question 3

1. Regardless of present residence, does this patient need skilled nursing services *in an institutional setting* (such as a nursing home, extended care facility, rehabilitation hospital, mental hospital)?

    yes_____   no_____

    If "Yes" is checked at right, *list nursing services needed.*

    _____

    _____

    _____

2a. Regardless of present residence, is this patient able to reside *in a residential setting* (such as patient's own home, relative or friend's home, hotel, or state licensed permit home)?

    yes_____   no_____

 b. Who is the person *who helps the patient most* in the residential setting? (Use your *best judgment* and any information you have from the patient or family to answer this question.)

    1. _____ a relative (specify relationship) _____

    2. _____ a friend or neighbor of the patient

    3. _____ an employee of the patient or patient's family

    4. _____ a nurse or other health service worker

    5. _____ some other type of person (specify) _____

 c. What is the name, address and phone number of the person checked in 2b? (Be as specific as you can, with the information available to you. Leave address and phone spaces blank, *if the address is the same as the address and phone at left.*)

Mr. Mrs. Miss
_____
      (last name)   (first name)

_____
(*Street & Number*, if dfferent from patient's)

_____
(*City & Phone*, if different from patient's)

113

d. If "yes" is checked for 2a., list the services needed by the patient, regardless of who provides the services in the residential setting.

_____

_____

_____

3. How would you describe the address at left?

1. _____ This is an institutional setting

2. _____ This is a residential setting

Appendix B

INTERVIEW SCHEDULE

PRIMARY PARTICIPANT
SECOND (6-MONTH) FOLLOW-UP INTERVIEW

Best Present Information: Home Address

Street _____

City _____ Zip _____ Telephone _____

Best Present Information: Primary Care Giver   Age _____ Sex _____

Name (PCG) _____ CDM # _____

Street _____ Relationship _____

City _____ Zip _____ Telephone _____

Starting Time of Interview _____

Others Present During Interview

Name	Role	Length of Time				
		All	M.	½	¼	Sh.

Delay During Interview

Reason for Delay	From:	To:	Minutes	Total Mins.

Record of Interview Attempts

APPOINTMENT ARRANGEMENTS					OUTCOME			REASON
Date	Time	Place	Arranged with (name)	Role	Complete	Refusal	Delay	GIVEN

117

NAME _____ AGE _____ SEX _____ CDM # _____

1. Since I talked with you last (during the last six months) have you been a patient in a hospital, nursing home or other such institution?
    1. Yes (ask item 2)
    2. No (skip item 2 and go to item 3)

2. What was the name of the place (places) where you were a patient? What month were you admitted? (After each stay has been recorded ask:)

Were you a patient in *any other* place during the last six months?

Name of Institution (List each stay in the order mentioned)	Hosp. ACF*	NH* ECF	Month	From ACF or ECF Records—Date of: Admission	Discharge

* Field Code as either Hospital or Acute Care Facility *OR* Nursing Home or Extended Care Facility (include Rehabilitation Hospital). If you do not know what the institution is from the name given, ask is that a hospital, nursing home, or what?

3. How long have you lived in your present home?
    2. Less than a month
    3. Less than a year
    4. At least 1 year, less than 5 years
    5. At least 5 years, less than 10 years
    6. 10 years or more
    9. No codable answer given

4. What is your address? (Do not ask if interview is at residence. Allow sufficient time for an unprompted response, before you mention the address supplied on page 1. Verify the address which has been given to you.)

    _____

    _____

5. What kind of place are you living in? Is it your own (or spouse's) home, someone else's home, or some other kind of place?
    1. My own or spouse's home
    2. Someone else's home

    3. A permit home
    4. A hotel or boarding home
    . First specific ECF in area
    . Second specific ECF in area
    . An acute care facility or hospital
    . Some other rehabilitation hospital, nursing home, ECF, or mental institution
    . Any setting (as a class) to which the interviewer cannot obtain entrance

6. How many other people live with you?

7. Who lives with you? (Table relationship & sex below)

8. How old are they? (Table age below)

9. Who is the head of the household or family? (Circle number below)

10. Who in your household works for money? (place X in "employed" space below) Are you employed for money or profit from your work (Even 1 hour a month)? (Record answer in row 7 below.)

11. Which of these persons works full time? (place x in "full time" space below)

	Relationship to Participant	Sex M F	Age	Employed	Full Time
1.					
2.					
3.					
4.					
5.					
6.					
7.	Self				
8.	Question skipped by RI				
9.	No codable answer given				

12. Who owns this place you're living in?
    1. No one who lives here—residence is rented from others by self or spouse or others who live here

2. Self or spouse own the home
3. Someone else who lives here owns the home
9. No codable answer given

13. Do you (or your spouse) own any residences or property *other than the place you live in?*
     1. At least 1 other residence I (we) have lived in previously
     2. At least 1 residence I (we) have never lived in
     3. Other types of property
     4. No *other* property is owned by the participant (or spouse)
     5. No property is owned by the participant (or spouse)
     9. No codable answer given

14. During the last six months have you lived at any other location than this address (not including the hospital stays we have just talked about)? (Even for a short time?)
     1. Yes (ask item 15)
     2. No (skip item 15 and go to item 15a)

15. Where was that? Did you pay for care while there? (Interviewer write some place description for each place mentioned, circle 1, 2, 3, 4 or 5 in each row, according to the following code, and check either "yes" or "no" in the paid column.)
     1. My own or spouses' home
     2. Someone else's home
     3. A permit home
     4. A hotel or boarding home
     5. "Other" type of residence

Did you live in *any other* location during the past 6 months, even for a short time?

Name of Place	# Code	Paid Yes	No	Name of Place	# Code	Paid Yes	No
	1 2 3 4 5				1 2 3 4 5		
	1 2 3 4 5				1 2 3 4 5		
	1 2 3 4 5				1 2 3 4 5		

15a. During the last six months has anyone important (close) to you moved away, so that it is inconvenient or impossible for you to get together? (neighbor, friend, relative, etc.)

1. Yes (Specify) _____ if more than one,
2. No   N = _____

15b. Are you employed for money or profit from your work? (even 1 hour a month) (if "no") Did you retire from your job (become unemployed) during the last six months? (If participant is getting sick leave pay they are still employed.)

    1. Yes—still employed (even 1 hour a month, or on sick leave)
    2. No—retired more than six months ago
    3. No—retired or stopped working for pay, but began to work again
    4. Never held a job for pay
    5. No—retired or stopped working for pay during the last six months

15c. During the last six months have you turned the household chores over to someone else? (Stopped doing household chores?)

    1. No—stopped doing housework (chores) more than six months ago
    2. No—still do the housework (chores
    3. Yes—stopped doing housework (majority of it) in last six months
    4. Yes—stopped doing housework, but began doing housework again
    5. Never did any (very much) housework or chores

15d. Are you married, divorced, widowed, separated (intentionally), or have you never married? (Note: Married takes precedence over *also* being divorced or widowed)

    1. Married (spouse may be separated for other reasons, such as hospitalization, military service, etc.)
    2. Divorced or separated (intentionally)
    3. Widowed
    4. Never married

15e. Has anyone important (close) to you passed away during the last six months?

    1. Yes (Specify) _____ If more than one,
    2. No   N = _____

15f. (If spouse has died in the last six months ask:) When did your wife/husband pass away?

    1. Spouse deceased in last six months (specify date) __/__/__
    2. Spouse still alive
    3. Never married

4. Divorced, separated (intentionally) or widowed more than 6 months ago

5. RI unable to determine

15i. Who is the person who gives you the most direct help with personal care and household tasks? (Probe: Things like bathing, dressing, laundry, cooking, shopping, cleaning, and such?) What is this person's relation to you?

1. Spouse
2. Other relative (Specify) _____
3. Friend
4. Neighbor
5. Employee
6. Other (Specify) _____

15j. (Ask only if the above named person does not live with participant) What is this person's name, address, and telephone number (If questioned add, Part of the research involves interviewing this person you've mentioned also.)

Address: Age _____ Sex _____

_____ Telephone _____

_____ (verify PCG address given on page 1)

16. During the past two weeks how many days did you stay in bed all or most of the day?

<u>(Number of days)</u>

17. Would you say that during the past two weeks you were able to do *many things, a few things, or nothing,* with your husband (wife)? (Table answer below)

18. Would you say that during the past two weeks you were able to do *many things, a few things, or nothing,* with your other relatives? (Table answer below)

19. Would you say that during the past two weeks you were able to do *many things, a few things, or nothing,* with your friends? (Table answer below)

20. Would you say that during the past two weeks you were able to work *full time, part time, or not at all* at your job? (Employment for pay, or housework, if that is person's occupation) (Table answer below)

(Mention of *any* contact, i.e. phone call or visit should be recorded as "a few things")

	Many things (full time)	*A few* things (part time)	*Nothing* (not at all)	DOESN'T APPLY *I have no such relation*	No Codable Answer
Spouse					
Other Relatives					
Friends					
Work (for pay)					
Housework					

26. Has your health been a worry for you during the past two weeks?
    1. No-unqualified
    2. Any answer which indicates some worry
    3. No codable answer

29. In general, how satisfied are you with your arrangements for housecleaning, cooking, laundry and shopping? *Are you satisfied, partly satisfied, or dissatisfied?* (Be sure to read the *choices* to the respondent)
    1. Satisfied (include "I have to be satisfied")
    2. Partly satisfied
    3. Dissatisfied
    9. No codable answer

(In the following ten items remember we are interested in what a person actually does, not what they feel they can do. Code the most dependent level in the past two weeks.)

33. Are you managing most of your personal care by yourself? For instance, do you take a bath in tub, in shower, or in bed? Does anyone help you to get in and out of the bathtub or shower? (In the past two weeks) (Probe: How do you bathe—in a shower? tub? or sponge bath? Does anyone help you bathe? If yes—Do you get help with only a single part or more than that? Does anyone go with you to your bath? Does anyone bring you your bath water?
    1. *Independent*
        a. bathes self completely, in shower, tub, or sponge bath
        b. gets assistance, support or supervision in bathing a single part (such as back or disabled extremity), or
    2. Dependent
        a. gets assistance, support or supervision in bathing more than one part of the body, or

       b.   gets assistance, support or supervision getting in and out of the tub, or to the bath

       c.   has bath water brought to them

       d.   does not bathe self

    7.   Refusal

    9.   No codable answer

34.   Do you get dressed every day? How do you manage your dressing? (in the past two weeks?) (Probe: Does anyone help you get your clothing out of closets and drawers? Does anyone help you get dressed?)

    1.   *Independent*

       a.   gets clothes from closets and drawers *and*

       b.   puts on brace every day (if necessary), and

       c.   puts on clothes, outer garments, stockings and shoes or slippers, and manages all clothing fasteners (except tying shoes, or zipping back zippers which is not necessary for an "independent" code)

    2.   *Dependent*

       a.   receives assistance or supervision in getting clothing out of closets and drawers *or*

       b.   receives assistance or supervision in getting dressed *or*

       c.   does not change attire (i.e. remains partly undressed e.g. shoes off, in bathrobe over pajamas)

    7.   Refusal

    9.   No codable answer

35.   How about toileting? (in past two weeks?) (Probe: How do you get to the bathroom? Does anyone help you with your toileting— help you with getting on the seat, with arranging your clothing, with cleaning yourself (private parts)? Do you use a bed pan or commode? Who empties it?)

    1.   *Independent*

       a.   gets to toilet room, *and*

       b.   gets on and off toilet, *and*

       c.   arranges clothes; cleans organs of excretion, *or*

       d.   may manage own bedpan or commode *at night only and empties it*

       e.   Note: it is acceptable for P to use mechanical supports such as cane, crutches, walkers, wheelchairs, etc.

    2.   *Dependent*

       a.   uses bedpan or commode during daytime, or uses either at night, *without emptying* it, *or*

    b. receives assistance or supervision in getting to toilet room, *or*

    c. receives assistance or supervision in getting on and off toilet seat, *or*

    d. receives assistance or supervision in arranging clothes, *or* cleaning organs of excretion

  7. Refusal

  9. No codable answer

36. Do you receive any help in eating? (in past two weeks)

  1. *Independent*

    a. gets food from plate (or its equivalent) into mouth

    b. note: not necessary that usual implements be used by P.

    c. note: acceptable to code as 1, independent, if the participant receives assistance in preparation of food, such as precutting of meat and buttering of bread.

  2. *Dependent*

    a. assistance given by other in act of feeding *or*

    b. does not eat at all—reliant on intraveneous feeding

  7. Refusal

  9. No codable answer

37. Do certain foods seem to give you problems with elimination? (in past two weeks) Do you have accidents with diarrhea? Do you *lose control* of your bowels or bladder? Do you have *accidents?*

  1. *Independent*

    a. urination and defecation entirely self-controlled, either by internal control or external management such as enemas, suppositories, colostomy, bedpan, urinal, etc.

  2. *Dependent*

    a. partial or total incontinence in urination or defecation or both *or*

    b. partial or total assistance or supervision of control by enemas, catheters, or use of urinals and/or bedpans, or colostomy

  7. Refusal

  9. No codable answer

38. Do you get in and out of bed by yourself (and/or in and out of chairs?) (in past two weeks) (Probe: How do you get out of bed? How do you get out of chairs?)

  11. Independent—Moves in and out of bed and chairs independently (Note: *artificial limbs* are not to be coded as a mechanical support)

12. Independent—Moves in or out of bed and chair using mechanical supports such as canes, crutches, walkers, wheelchairs, etc. but without help from another person

23. Dependent—has assistance of another person for moving in and out of bed or chair, but uses no mechanical devices

24. Dependent—has assistance from another person and from mechanical devices for moving in and out of bed or chair

25. Dependent—Another person carries participant from bed or chair, participant does not participate in the activity

26. Dependent—Participant does not leave bed

39. Do you walk by yourself (in past two weeks) (Probe: Do you use anything to help you walk (Includes handrails or furniture, if that is the only way the person can walk inside the house.) Does anyone help you walk?)

1. Independent—walks without help from other person or any devices (Note: *artificial limbs* are not to be coded as a mechanical support)

2. Walks only using mechanical supports (cane, crutches, walker, wheelchair, braces) but without help from another person

3. Walks with the assistance of another person, but without any mechanical devices (assistance may include visual supervision of another person if the participant does not walk until the other person is overseeing the activity

4. Walks with assistance from another person and mechanical devices (example: uses cane on one side, other person on other side)

5. Does not move about—another person carries participant. Participant does not take part in moving activity

6. Does not walk—does not move from bed

40. (Ask only if person has mentioned a wheelchair, or if you see a wheelchair) Do you use your wheelchair (cart) by yourself? (In past two weeks) (Probe: Do you wheel through doorways, up ramps, and lock and unlock the brakes yourself? Does someone push the chair, or is it electric? Do you need any special equipment so you can wheel yourself?)

1. Independent—Wheels without any help from persons or devices

2. Uses electric wheelchair, amputee or one-arm drive wheelchair but wheels without help of any other person

3. Wheels with help of another person, but participant does take part in the wheeling activity. No devices are used other than the wheelchair.

    4. Wheels with help of another person and some special devices or equipment. Participant takes some part in the wheeling activity.

    5. Someone else wheels the participant. Participant takes no part in the wheeling activity.

    6. Is not wheeled—bedfast or chairfast.

    8. Does not apply—person not in need of using wheeled device.

41. Do you go up and down stairs by yourself? (in past two weeks) (Probe: Does anyone help you, or do you use specially placed stair rails?)

    1. Independent—goes up and down stairs with no special devices, crutches, canes, etc. and without any other person's help. (need not be upright)

    2. Uses canes, crutches, special handrails, but without other person's help to go up and down stairs

    3. Goes up and down stairs with other person's help, but without the help of any special devices

    4. Goes up and down stairs with another person's help, and with the help of some special devices

    5. Does not participate in going up and down stairs, is carried by another person

    6. Does not go up and down stairs—is bound to the floor (story) they're on. May use an elevator. May be able to go up and down 1 step (curb).

42. Do you go outside of the building by yourself? (In past two weeks) (Probe: Does anyone help you or purposely accompany you? Do you use any special devices when you go outside of the building?)

    1. Independent—Goes outside of building without any special devices, or the help or accompaniment of any other person

    2. Uses cane, crutches, walker, wheelchair, or other special devices, but without the help of another person to go outside of the building

    3. Uses help or accompaniment of another person but no devices to move outside of the building

    4. Uses help or accompaniment of another person and special devices to move outside of the building

    5. Does not participate in going outside of the building. Is carried outside by another person

    6. Does not go outside of the building. Confined to house.

43. Would you say that you have been happy or unhappy during these past two weeks?
    1. Happy
    2. Both happy and unhappy
    3. Unhappy
    9. No codable answer given

44. In general how satisfied are you with your way of life today? *Are you satisfied, partly satisfied, or dissatisfied?* (Be sure to read the *choices* to participant)
    1. Satisfied
    2. Partly satisfied
    3. Dissatisfied
    9. No codable answer given

45. Would you agree or disagree with those people who say, "Things just keep getting worse for me as I get older"?
    1. Agree
    2. Disagree
    3. No codable answer given

46. During the last month did you receive any help in your home from any friends or relatives who do not live with you? (Not just social visiting.)
    1. No—(skip item 47 and go to item 50)
    2. Yes—(specify number of persons during the month, and ask item 47.) _____

47. What kinds of things have these friends or relatives (who do not live with you) helped you with during the last month? (Circle any numbers which participant *mentions*.)
    1. Laundry
    2. Meal or food preparation (includes dishes)
    3. Making up the bed
    4. Housecleaning
    5. Shopping
    6. Transporation of participant
    7. Any other help (specify _____
    8. Not asked by RI

50. Would you say your health is better, the same, or worse than when I last talked to you, six months ago?
    1. Better
    2. The same
    3. Worse
    9. Don't know

51. We're interested in knowing how long your health has been like it is right now. How long have you needed the kind of help you need at present? (Probe: How long has your health been like it is at present?)

    1. More than two years (1½ years before initial interview)
    2. More than a year (6 months before initial interview)
    3. More than six months
    4. More than five months
    5. More than four months
    6. More than three months
    7. More than two months
    8. More than a month
    9. A month or less
    0. Don't need any help (ask probe).

52. How many months or weeks has it been since a doctor (M.D. or D.O.) last examined or talked to you? (Count "today" or "less than a week" as one week.)

    _____ months, _____ weeks (specify numbers)
    98. Don't know
    99. No codable answer

53. Where did this last contact with a doctor occur?

    1. In my home
    2. In a doctor's office
    3. In a clinic (several doctors)
    4. In a hospital (ACF)
    5. On the telephone
    7. Other (specify) _____
    8. Not asked by RI
    9. No codable answer or don't know

54. Do you have a regular doctor? (either M.D. or D.O.)

    1. Yes
    2. No
    3. Refusal
    9. No codable answer

55. What would you estimate was your total health care bill *for the past month*? (Only include costs for participant's health care, and not for other household members' health care in this estimate.) Try to think of all your costs for doctors, other health care workers, medicines, and any special equipment which you need, plus your hospital (nursing home) bill. (Attempt to learn if participant did or did not have health care costs in the last month. If they did not have such costs enter "0" in the estimate space.

If they did have such costs—do your best to obtain the best estimate of the amount. Use the "Don't know" box only as a last resort.)

Don't know __   Enter estimate _____

(If no institutions are listed in table for item 2, page 3, skip item 55a below.)

55a.   How much (money) has your hospital (nursing home) bill come to during the past month? (record in table below, for one or two separate stays in a hospital or nursing home during the past month. Include charges for the operating room, anesthesia, x-rays, tests, special treatments, etc.)

	Amount of Bill
Hospital, Nursing Home Bill—Present Stay	
Hospital, Nursing Home Bill—Earlier Stay	

56.   How many times in the last month has your doctor examined or talked to you? (Enter your answers in the first column of the table below. Record a "0" where it is appropriate.)

57.   How many times in the last month has any other type of doctor examined or talked to you, such as a dentist, an eye doctor, a foot doctor, a psychiatrist, or any other?

(If responses to items 56 and 57 are "none," enter "0" on table and skip to item 61.)

58.   Was the charge for the _____ charged on your hospital (nursing home) bill? (Distinguish between staff whose services are included in the H/NH bills, and other physicians, such as specialists or the patient's private physician, whose charges are in addition to the H/NH bill. Record a charge only for those doctors who render a bill additional to the H/NH bill. If charge for doctor is included on H/NH bill, place an "X" in the H/NH column on table below.)

59.   What was the charge for the services of the _____ during the last month? We are interested in knowing the charge made by the doctor, even if you did not pay the full fee yourself. (Estimate if necessary. Probe: Did you receive a bill? How much was it for?) (Repeat this wording of the question for each professional who was seen at least once during the last month, and not charged on the H/NH bill. Do not record charges included on institution

billings and recorded in item 55a. If charge for doctor is included on H/NH bill, leave "charge" column blank on table below.)

(Take care that you do not appear "eager" to look at bills and personal papers of the respondent. Only if bills or other papers are proffered to you willingly should you look at them. Do not ask to look at such papers. In any situation where you are shown bills, *try to look at them without handling* the papers themselves. If the participant asks you to get papers from some distant part of the room or residence, do so without looking at them until after the participant has shown them to you.)

(For all items which ask for a "charge" or "amount of bill" estimate total bill, regardless of how much the patient has paid and regardless of what sources may have paid for part of the bill.)

Record answers to 56, 57, 58, and 59 below

	HOW MANY TIMES?	H/NH BILL	WHAT WAS THE COST?
Your Doctor (any M.D. or D.O. seen in last month, if has no regular doctor)			
A Dentist			
An Eye Doctor (Ophthalmologist, Optometrist, Optician, Oculist Do not limit to M.D. only)			
A Foot Doctor (Chiropodist)			
A Psychiatrist (Clinical Psychologist)			
Any other (Specialists, etc.) Specify _____			
Subtotal A (Medical Services)			

(Excuse yourself and take the time to total first and third columns. Carry these totals, and the amounts of the hospital bills forward to the designated spaces in the table on page 13)

61. How many times in the last month have registered nurses seen you or talked to you (outside of a doctor's office)? (This does not include social contacts with nurses who are relatives, friends, or acquaintances of the participant. Enter your answers in the first column of the table below. Record "0" when appropriate. Make entry regardless of whether the health care provider was seen in an institution, residence, or elsewhere. If more than one R.N. was seen during the past month enter total number of times for all R.N.'s in this column.)

62. How many times in the last month have any other types of health workers seen you or talked to you (outside of a doctor's office): such as L.P.N.'s, nurse's aides, housekeepers (presence due to participant's health), social workers, physical therapists, occupational therapists, or any others? (Enter your answers in the first column of the table below.)

(If responses to items 61 and 62 are "none," enter "0" and skip to item 66 below.)

63. Did you see the _____ in your home or elsewhere? (Repeat this form of the question for each health care provider who was seen at least once during the last month. Record "here" answers with an "X" in the "in home" column of the following table. If answer refers to an inpatient facility record an "X" in the "in inst." column.)

64. How many hours of service did you receive from the _____ in the past month? (What is your best guess at the average number of hours?) (Repeat this form of the question for each type of health care provider who was seen at least once during the last month. Record some answer for each type in the "how many hours" column of the following table. If the health care provider lives in the home, write "li" in the hours column.)

64a. Was the charge for the _____ charged on your hospital (nursing home) bill? (Distinguish between health care providers whose services are included in the H/NH bill and other health care providers whose charges would be on a separate billing, such as private duty nurses. Record a charge only for those health care providers who render a bill additional to the H/NH bill. If charge for health care provider is included on H/NH bill, place an "X" in the H/NH column in table below.)

65. What was the charge for the services of the _____ during the last month? We are interested in knowing the charge made, even if you did not pay the full fee yourself. (Estimate if necessary.) Probe: Did you receive a bill? How much was it for? (Repeat this wording of the question for each health care provider who was seen at least once during the last month and not charged on the H/NH bill. Do not record charges included on institution billings and recorded in item 55a. If charge for health care provider is included on H/NH bill leave "charge" column blank on table below.)

66. Were there any additional charges (full charges) for your health care during the last month? We are interested in knowing the charge made, even if you did not pay the full fee yourself. (Do

not include anything already accounted for. Some examples are: Things such as medicines, special equipment, wheelchairs, beds, glasses, hearing aid, etc. Enter a total on the line for "additional charges" in second table below.)

Record answers to 61, 62, 63, 64a, 65, and 55a below.

	How many times?	In inst.	In home	How many hours?	H/NH bill	What was the charge?
Registered Nurses (R.N.'s)						
Licensed Practical Nurses (L.P.N.'s)						
Nurse's Aides						
Housekeepers (presence in home due to participant's health)						
Social Workers						
Physical Therapists						
Occupational Therapists						
Other Health Care Providers Specify _____						
Subtotal B (Health Care Providers)						
Subtotal A (enter from page)	(Excuse yourself and take the time to total columns for Subtotals B, C, and Total)					___
Hospital Bill—Most Recent						
Stay (Enter from item 55a)						___
Subtotal C (Enter from below)						___
Total Health Care Costs						___

Record Answers to Item 66 Below

Additional Charges (specify below)	Charge
Medicines (#1)	
Other Charge #2	
Other Charge #3	
Other Charge #4	
Additional Costs—Subtotal C	

67. (Refer to item 55. Enter estimate from that source.) _____
(If total obtained in total of table above is as much as 20% less than the amount recorded here ask the following item. Otherwise continue with item 68.) Earlier you estimated your total health

care bill for last month as _____ is there anything (any charge) we haven't included in the total I have? (Make adjustments in tables or item 55 as necessary.)

68. During the past six months was anyone in your family, or anyone who lives here with you, prevented from working because they have been giving you care?

    1. No—(Skip item 69 and go to item 71).
    2. Yes—(Specify relationship) _____
    9. Don't know or not sure

69. How long has _____ been giving you care which made it necessary that he/she not work for pay?

    Years, _____ Months, _____ Weeks, _____ Days, _____ (specify number(s))

71. Let me read you a list of sources of income. From which of these did you (or your spouse) receive your income in the last six months? (Circle as many codes as apply)

    1. During the last six months did you (or your spouse) receive any income from *salary, wages or commission*? (Even if only 1 hour's work per month) (Also payment for any product of the participant's industry which results in a profit. Includes any "sick pay" in income)
    2. During the last six months did you (or your spouse) receive any income from *social security payments*? (Does not include SSI payments)
    3. During the last six months did you (or your spouse) receive any income from *public assistance*? (Aid to the Aged, Aid for the Blind, Aid for the Disabled, Welfare payments of any kind, Unemployment Compensation, SSI payments from Social Security)
    4. During the last six months did you (or your spouse) receive any income from *pensions or retirement funds*? (Derived from own or spouse's past employment or savings, such as: Veterans' Compensations, company pensions, retirement plans, Workman's Compensation, etc.)
    5. During the last six months did you (or your spouse) receive any income from *paid up annuities, insurance, interest, dividends, rentals, etc.*? (Continuing income from a previous investment)
    6. During the last six months did you (or your spouse) receive any income from *withdrawals from savings, cashing bonds,*

selling things you own? (One time income from a previous investment)

7. During the last six months did you (or your spouse) receive any income from *gifts from children, relatives, friends, or private social agencies?*
0. During the last six months did you (or your spouse) receive any income from *loans from any source?*
8. Question skipped by RI
9. No codable answer
10. No income

73. Now I'd like to read (show) you a table of levels of income and have you tell me the level that comes closest to the combined total income for you and all those persons who live with you and are also related to you by blood, marriage, or adoption. (These are only broad ranges of income. We don't need the specific amount of your income.) Please think of the total income for the past 12 months before any taxes or other deductions were taken out. (Think about all the possible sources of income I've just mentioned.)

	Per Year	*Per Month*	*Per Week*
1.	Less than $3,000	Less than $250	Less than $60
2.	$3,000 to $4,999	$250 to $416	$60 to $99
3.	$5,000 to $6,999	$417 to $583	$100 to $139
4.	$7,000 to $9,999	$584 to $833	$140 to $199
5.	$10,000 to $14,999	$834 to $1,249	$200 to $299
6.	More than $14,999	More than $1,249	More than $299

(If no health care costs have been mentioned by participant, skip items 74 and 75.)

74. Let me read you a list of sources of payment for health care. From which of these did (or will) you or your spouse pay for your personal health care (your hospital bill, nursing home bill) during the last month? (Probe: Who will pay, even if you will not receive a bill?) (Circle as many codes as apply below. Health care for participant only, does not include health care for spouse.)

1. *Private Health Insurance* (Blue Cross, Blue Shield, employee or union health benefits, Workman's Compensation, Veteran's Compensation, etc.)
2. *Medicare*
3. *Medicaid*

4. *Public Assistance* (Other forms, such as Aid for Aged, State Social Services, Aid for the Blind, Aid for the Disabled, Unemployment Compensation, Welfare payments of any kind)

5. *Your own (or spouse's) money* (through salary, other income, savings, borrowed money or Social Security)

6. *Family or friends* (through gifts, not loans to you. Probe: Do you expect to pay that money back?)

7. Other sources (Specify) _____

75. Of the different sources we've been talking about, which one did (or will) pay the largest part of the costs of your health care (your hospital bill, nursing home bill) during the past month?

(Specify Source) _____

Now here are some questions we need to ask everyone.

76. What is the date today? _____

77. (ask only if not given in answer to "76" above) What month is it now? _____

78. What year is it now? _____

79. How old are you? _____

80. What month were you born? _____

81. What year were you born? _____

82. What is the name of this place? (Probe: What do you call this place?) (Write out address, street, name of apartment complex, hotel, housing unit, etc.) _____

83. (Ask only if address not given in answer to "82" above) Where is it located? (Write out city, street or address given.) _____

84. Who is President of the United States? _____

85. Who was President before him? _____

Now this is a somewhat different thing I'm going to have you do

(For participant who appears mentally alert, and physically able) I'm going to ask you to go through the pages of this booklet and mark the correct choices on this sheet. (Don't pay any attention to the paper clips.) (You may help participant by turning the pages.)

(For participant who appears mentally alert but physically unable or unwilling to write) I'm going to ask you to go through the pages of this booklet and tell me the correct choice for each page. (Don't pay any attention to the paper clips) (You must have them tell you the number of the problem before each answer choice, or you must visually verify that they are at the right page of the book. They may turn two pages at once. If this happens early in the test, all their answers will be in error. If they come out with one more or less answer than there are answer spaces, try again.)

(For all other participants) I'm going to ask you to look at each of the pictures I show you, and decide which of the pieces completes the picture.

Standard directions for picture A1

Look here (Point finger at edge of upper picture). This is a picture of a pattern (design) with a piece cut out of it. Each of these pieces (Point to each of the six pieces in turn) is the right shape to fit the space. (Use finger to go around the outline of figure 2., the plain green piece. Then put your finger inside of the missing space in the upper figure) Only one of these pieces is the right pattern (design) to make the picture complete. Point to the one piece which is right (tell me which one piece is right). Take as much time to decide as you need. Be careful, look at each piece before you decide. You may change your mind if you feel you need to.

(After each choice is made, accept the choice with approval, such as an up and down nod of the head, or okay/ all right/ fine/ go on/ go right ahead/ good/ uh huh/ yes/ I've got that answer, etc. Record the number of each answer in the recording space. If you think an answer is wrong, give no hint of this to the participant. Keep moving right along. *Do not give a positive response to a participant who fails to respond with a definite choice.* Probe: You must choose only one. Remember, only one is right. Which one of the pieces completes the picture? Point to the one piece which came out of this picture (pattern). Take as much time as you need, but be sure to choose just one of the pieces.)

Standard directions for picture Ab1

It's all right to take as much time as you need. Be sure to look at the picture of the pattern (design). Make certain you look at all six pieces before you make your choice.

Standard directions for picture B1

Remember to look at the picture to see what part of the design is missing. Then look at each piece to see which one came out of this picture. Take as much time as you need.

A1	Ab1	B1
A3	Ab3	B3
A5	Ab5	B5
A7	Ab7	B7
A9	Ab9	B9
A11	Ab11	B11

Thank you very much for your time.
We really appreciate your help with   Ending Time _____
this research. Good-bye for now.
(If possible, check over interview for
completeness before leaving.)

INDEX